A HEALTHY STATE

A
Healthy State

An International
Perspective
on the Crisis
in United States
Medical Care

by Victor W. Sidel and Ruth Sidel

Pantheon Books, New York

Library of Congress Cataloging in Publication Data

Sidel, Victor W.
    A Healthy State.

    Includes bibliographical references and index.
    1. Medical care—United States.   I.   Sidel, Ruth,
joint author. II.   Title. [DNLM: 1. Delivery of
health care. 2. Delivery of health care—United
States. 3. Health sevices. 4. Health services—
United States. W84 AA1 S516h]
RA395.A3S52   362.1′0973   77–5196
ISBN 0–394–40760–1

Grateful acknowledgment is made to the following for permission to reprint previously
published material:

Department of Medical Care Organization, School of Public Health, The University of Michigan: Figures 8, 11, and 12 appearing in the *Medical Chart Book*,
6th Edition, September, 1976.

Neale Watson Academic Publications, Inc.: Figure 14 from *Medicine Under
Capitalism* by Vincent Navarro. Copyright © 1976 by Neale Watson Academic
Publications, Inc.

For
Dr. Salvador Allende Gossens
and the other health workers of Chile
who were killed or are in exile
because they knew that the only way
to protect and promote the health of a nation
is to redistribute wealth and power among its people

"El pueblo unido jamás será vencido."

ACKNOWLEDGMENTS

We are grateful to the many people who have helped in the writing of this book: To those who facilitated our visits to and our learning about their countries—in Sweden, Ragnar Berfenstam, Sixten Haraldson, Ake Lindgren, Bengt Mollstedt, Ake Norden, Bjorn Smedby, and Marianne Wistrand; in Great Britain, Stuart Carne, Ann Cartwright, John Fry, Donald Grant, John Horder, and Margot Jefferys; in the USSR, the Ministry of Health and particularly Deputy Minister Dmitri Venediktov; and in China, the Chinese Medical Association and Ma Hai-teh (George Hatem), Yang Ming-ting, Chang Wei-hsun, and particularly Hsu Chia-yu.

Among those who reviewed and commented on parts of the international section are Edgar Borgenhammar, Hugh Faulkner, Molly Coye, Roger Glass, Sixten Haraldson, Margot Jefferys, Bengt Mollstedt, Bjorn Smedby, and Patrick Storey. Those who reviewed and made comments on other parts of the manuscript include Daniel Drosness, Sandra Friedman, H. Jack Geiger, Daniel Lindheim, William Wilkinson, and Herbert Zollner. We particularly thank those who worked patiently through repeated drafts of the manuscript: Ruth Artig, Sharon Lockett, Jean Nardelli, Martha Russo, Eve Teitelbaum, and Phoebe Weber. We are grateful to Diana Perez, our copyeditor, and to Carol Lazare, at Pantheon Books, for their assistance.

Some of the material in Chapter 1 was originally gathered in collaboration with Steven Jonas for an article on the delivery of medical care in the United States. Some of the material in Chapter 6 is adapted from an article written with Robert Greifinger on the history of American medicine. We gratefully acknowledge their contributions.

Our recent visits to other countries and the analysis of their systems and of our own would not have been possible without the sustained encouragement of Martin Cherkasky and other colleagues at Montefiore Hospital; we are grateful to them.

We deeply appreciate the efforts of our editor, James Peck, who believed in the book and helped us at every stage. And finally, our gratitude to our sons, Mark and Kevin, for their support and, as the Chinese would say, their "revolutionary optimism."

CONTENTS

LIST OF FIGURES

LIST OF TABLES

A HEALTHY STATE

An International Perspective on the Crisis in United States Medical Care

INTRODUCTION

The word "crisis" is frequently used in discussions of the U.S. health-care and medical-care system. We too have used it, but to us it has a special meaning. The Chinese character for "crisis" is made up of two different characters, one signifying "danger" and the other "opportunity." The dangers of American medicine, both of omission and of commission, have been widely discussed and many of them are documented in this book. What is less clear is the nature of the opportunity.

It is commonly accepted, and we concur, that fundamental change cannot be made from within the system; those to whom health care and medical care give profits, prestige and power will not willingly relinquish them. And a politically timid administration and Congress will hesitate to antagonize the powerful forces in medicine that defend the present system or at most offer stopgap measures which are designed to preserve its basic structure.

Fundamental change can come, however, from the mobilization of a political constituency which demands it. We believe that conditions in the U.S. health-care and medical-care system are such that this mobilization is not only clearly necessary but also possible.

How can such a political constituency be mobilized? Part of the strategy of those who control the American health-care and medical-care system has been to mystify, to obfuscate, to use the technical knowledge of the professional to retain the power to determine social policy. One way to mobilize the necessary constituency is through clear and forthright presentation to the American people of the problems and inequities that permeate American medicine. Another part of the strategy of those who seek to preserve the current system has been to narrow the options for discussion by disparaging the accomplishments of other systems. Thus an additional method of encouraging national debate and mobilizing forces for change is to widen the range of options for discussion. This requires the presentation of alternative models from other countries to indicate the spectrum of choices open to us.

This book is therefore intended for the general reader rather than the medical specialist. Our intention is to present some of the problems and some of the options, to provoke debate and discussion, but not to suggest simple solutions for complex problems. Our aim is, in short, to help to place the issue of health care and medical care for the American people into the political arena where decisions can be made, as they should be made in all major policy matters, by the people themselves.

In considering alternatives, it is often the view from outside one's society that is most enlightening. That which surrounds us, that which is most commonplace, is least likely to be noticed and least likely to be questioned. We may take much for granted, assume much is unchangeable, even satisfactory, which an outsider can tell us is very different elsewhere and can be different for us as well.

There are, for the United States, two centuries of precedents. One of the first was set by Alexis de Tocqueville, who analyzed both the successes and the failures of the United States with a clarity unavailable here. One of the more recent observers, the Swedish economist Gunnar Myrdal, analyzed race relations in the United States—and, more generally, some of the problems of justice, liberty and equality of opportunity—in *The American Dilemma*. He analyzed them so cogently that the U.S. Supreme Court used the analysis in its landmark decision declaring segregation in public education unconstitutional. In his most recent addresses to audiences at U.S. universities, Myrdal has expanded his analysis. He characterizes the United States as "that country among the rich countries that has the worst slums, the highest rate of unemployed and unemployable, and the least developed health services, and that is the most niggardly toward its old people and its poor children who are so many, as well as being the country that leads the whole Western world in violence, crime and corruption in high places."

But while Tocqueville, Myrdal, and many in between, have provided analyses uncommon in their perception and vision, all too often analysts from other societies, despite their advantage of perspective, face severe limitations in their analyses. They have rarely had the opportunity for in-depth study of the system they are analyzing, and therefore their analyses may in some ways be superficial, lacking in nuance and detail.

In this book we attempt, insofar as we can, to combine in an analysis of the U.S. health-care and medical-care system the advantages of the outsider's perspective and the insider's knowledge of nuance and detail, of both theoretical study and practical experience. We, as physician and social worker, have had the opportunity of working closely with others—colleagues and collaborators, patients and clients, students and teachers, friends and neighbors—in attempts to find short-term solutions to day-to-day problems in the United States. Yet we have also been fortunate in having had the chance to gain a longer-range perspective from outside our system. We have had opportunities to observe health care and medical care in other societies through formal study fellowships, exchange visitorships, WHO-sponsored and other consultantships, conferences, guided tours, lecture trips, and brief but professionally oriented visits. The countries in which we have had these opportunities include Argentina, Chile (during the Allende administration) and Colombia in South America; Denmark, Great Britain, Norway, Sweden and the USSR in Europe; and China, Malaysia, the Philippines and Vietnam (North Vietnam, while the war was still on) in Asia. From these experiences, both inside and outside the United States, we believe we can offer some insights into some of the critical problems the health-care and medical-care system in the United States is facing and some possible solutions.

As part of our attempt to clarify and propose remedies for problems within the United States, we will examine in this book the health-care and medical-care systems of four other countries—becoming in our turn "foreign" analysts with all of the liabilities and perhaps a few of the assets which accompany that task. The countries we have selected are Sweden, Great Britain, the Soviet Union and the People's Republic of China. These societies range from the highly urbanized to the predominantly rural; from a country with a population only slightly larger than that of the city of New York to the country with the world's largest population; from those with mixed economies, in which the private sector has significant and perhaps determining and overriding economic and political power, to those with virtually no private enterprise; from those that are highly centralized in their political organization to those that have made real efforts at decentralization. But what these four countries have in common is that each has made a significant effort to develop its health-care and medical-care system in a highly planned and organized way. Furthermore, in addition to attempting to maximize health and medical care for its people, each country has attempted to use the system to advance other social goals as well. These efforts are in important ways quite different from our own.

In looking at these other systems we will also briefly examine the historical roots of each system and attempt to trace its evolution. Our hope is that we in the United States can better analyze our own current medical dilemmas through an examination of how other societies have handled theirs. We recognize of course that transplantation of systems between societies with different historical roots and different societal structures is rarely possible, but the insights provided by markedly different approaches to the solution of comparable problems may be useful in our own search for solutions.

At this point a note on our use of the terms "health care" and "medical care" becomes necessary. Although health care and medical care overlap and intertwine in many ways, a clear and useful differentiation can be made between them. By "health care" we mean that part of the system which deals with the promotion and protection of health, including environmental protection, the protection of the individual in the workplace, the prevention of accidents, the provision of pure food and water, and other activities which are largely beyond the capability of the individual and must be done by the society as a whole. In addition there are many facets of health protection that are left largely to the individual—such as proper diet, care of one's body, and abstinence from voluntary use of substances known to be harmful.

In many areas, of course, there is overlap between societal responsibility and individual responsibility in health protection. Smoking is an example of such joint responsibility. While the individual must make the basic decision to abstain from smoking when cigarettes are available, society plays a considerable role in making them available and, more important, in permitting the glamorizing of smoking through vast advertising campaigns which promote the association of cigarettes with youth or sex, heighten peer pressure and thus induce people to begin smoking or to continue the habit. Blaming individuals for socially determined unhealthful habits—a form of "blaming the victim" increasingly being heard—is a way of avoiding the examination of society's responsibility. Society, as Norman Bethune has aptly said, often "makes the wounds" and it is part of the health-care system's responsibility to keep society from doing so.

Of course, much that promotes health and prevents disease has little to do with "health care" as it is conventionally defined. The level of food, clothing, shelter and living conditions undoubtedly has more to do with the level of health than do specific health-care measures. It has been convincingly demonstrated that, in England, deaths due to diseases such as diphtheria, tuberculosis and bronchitis began to decrease with change

in nutrition and other living conditions—long before the introduction of immunization, early detection or other specific prevention or treatment procedures. Indeed these developments,
when introduced, had relatively little effect on the already rapidly declining rate of deaths from these illnesses. The relative
impact of "health care" and social and environmental change
on other measures of health is harder to define, but social and
environmental change are almost certainly the more important
factors.

By "medical care" on the other hand, we mean that part of
the system which deals with individuals who are sick or who
think they may be sick (the "worried well"). Medical care must
have elements which provide reassurance for those who are
anxious or have self-limited illnesses for which no technical
care is required; elements which provide symptomatic relief and
emotional support for those whose illness will continue but
either need no further intervention or for whom further intervention would be useless or dangerous; elements which provide
appropriate skilled diagnosis and treatment for those patients
whose illnesses require it; elements which provide continuing
care and rehabilitation for patients with chronic illness and
disability; and elements which mobilize appropriate community resources for those who need them.

Clearly there is considerable overlap between what is called
"health care" and what is called "medical care." Health education, for example, is usually considered a part of health care, but
the occasion of medical care often serves as an opportunity for
effective transmittal of knowledge and skills or for helping to
change the patient's attitudes toward unhealthy habits. Another example of overlap is in the early detection of certain
illnesses, which often increases the chances of reversing or ar-
resting them; screening for such illnesses can either be provided
in the community as part of health care or can be done by the
physician or other health worker as part of what is usually
considered the work of medical care.

In prenatal care, for example, the borderline between what
is health care and what is medical care is a particularly hazy

one. Many obstetricians, highly trained in all of the possible complications which may occur during pregnancy and delivery, and clearly associated with the medical-care part of the system, often become frustrated and bored by the routine of caring for pregnant women, very few of whom will bring to the obstetrician a dreadful complication with which the obstetrician alone is equipped to deal. The protection of the health of pregnant women and their babies may be far better served by other types of health professionals, such as midwives—more appropriately perhaps considered members of the health-care part of the system—whose training and interest is predominantly in the promotion of the health of the woman and the baby rather than in dealing with the rare and difficult complication. Close interaction between the two elements, or better still a fusion of the two, is needed if both the majority of women with uncomplicated pregnancies and deliveries and the few women with complications are to be well served.

But profound tensions exist between the role of workers in health care and the role of workers in medical care or even within the work of a single individual or institution trying to do both. Physicians, public health nurses and other professionals associated primarily with the prevention of disease and protection of health frequently see themselves as educators, as promoters of the individual's understanding of and participation in his or her own health care, and as guardians of environmental conditions which will promote health rather than sickness. Professionals associated primarily with medical care, on the other hand, frequently function at times of crisis or emergency, when their patients are ill and anxious and when their task is primarily one of intervention, care and "healing," rather than teaching. While workers in health care often see the community as a whole as their responsibility, workers in medical care get caught up in the urgent "cases" which flood into their offices and hospitals day after day.

In short, although health care and medical care overlap in many ways and are often referred to together under the overall name of "health care" and even at times under the heading "medical care," we feel it important to maintain the conceptual distinction between the two in our analysis. This book is largely about *medical* care in the United States and other countries, but health care is so intertwined with it in all societies that it is usually impossible to talk of one without some discussion of the other, and much that we will say applies to both.

Furthermore, although some have argued that health care and medical care are so fragmented and so irrationally organized in the United States that they should be termed a "nonsystem," anyone who has ever tried to change it knows just how systematized, institutionalized and entrenched our health-care and medical-care system is. "System" also has a technical meaning, denoting the interdependence of its parts; and indeed, change in any part of the system, as the introduction of Medicare and Medicaid demonstrated, for example, has a profound effect on other parts of the system. We must therefore, regretfully, repeatedly use a tortuous phrase, "the health-care and medical-care system," when we want to refer to principles or observations that apply to it as a whole.

Before we proceed with an analysis of either our own system or that of others, we must state some basic assumptions concerning the purposes of the system which clearly color our perception of our experiences and determine our choice of recommendations. To illustrate the wide range of views on possible goals, let us consider some types of service provision other than health care and medical care.

The goal of an orchestra, for example, may to one observer —particularly if the observer is a musician or a conductor—be the brilliant rendition of fine music. To another observer the goal may lie in the orchestra's effect on its audience, be it contentment, excitement or the desire to move mountains. To yet another the goal of an orchestra may lie in the number of people it reaches with its music. Some, on the other hand, may judge it by the number of jobs it creates for musicians and others. For some observers the critical question may be whether those the orchestra reaches and those it employs lack other opportunities for listening to music or for productive employment, so that the opportunities the orchestra provides are an important factor in the redistribution of resources. The manager, the conductor or the musician as participants, the musician or nonmusician as listeners, the affluent and the poor, the "conservative," the "liberal" and the "radical" are likely to have different views of the purposes of an orchestra and therefore different views of how well it performs its tasks.

It would appear that the goals of a plumbing company, to take another example, might be easier to define. Yet some of the different ways of looking at the goals of a plumbing company are remarkably analogous: *e.g.*, technical skill and performance, functional outcome of work, satisfaction of clients (which may be based as much on the attitude of the workers as on the outcome of their work), accessibility of services to those in need, and provision of employment.

Both examples suggest that each observer's, user's or provider's definition of the purpose of a service depends at root on his or her view of the nature of society and its purposes, and on his or her own place in it, as well as, more narrowly, on his or her role in relation to the service. Basic questions about society and its services lie behind the definitions of purpose: For whom are services to be provided? To what end are they given? More specifically and more importantly: Are the services directed toward those who already have much or toward those who have relatively little? Are the services directed toward redressing this imbalance or do they, in effect if not in conscious design, widen the existing gap between those who are wealthy and those who are poor? Do they strengthen individual, family and community life, or weaken it?

Health care and medical care, like other services, are a means to an end, rather than an end in themselves. What then are *our* views on the ends of a health-care and medical-care system? What are *our* answers to the questions "For whom?" and "To what purpose?"

1. We believe that the most fundamental purpose of social institutions is that of justice—justice in its Aristotelian sense: a fair distribution of all that is of value in society. It is a goal

that has also in some contexts been termed "equity." Furthermore we believe that the assumption that justice or equity for everyone is society's fundamental purpose leads inexorably to the conclusion that the improvement of life for those who have least—rather than increased power, wealth or consumption for those who have most—must be the society's highest priority. We see equity as a fundamental goal not only in the narrow interpretation of equity of access to services, as the goal is often expressed in discussions of medical care, but also in the sense of control of resources, work satisfaction and the power to shape one's environment. Without equity in this broader sense, we feel, equity of access to health- and medical-care services is not only impossible to attain but even meaningless.

Lest the goal of equity and justice seem absurd in a competitive, individualistic society such as the United States, it should be pointed out that the idea of equity is deeply ingrained in our society. We would argue that there is a fundamental egalitarian, antielitest stream which runs through American history, which can be developed and fostered. Its most obvious manifestation is in the "one man, one vote" concept. There are many societies, past and present, which reject even such a limited idea of equity, yet it is one to which most people in the United States would at least pay lip service. Another example of a commitment to equity in the United States is support—though surely inconsistent at times—of a universal right to education. Over 90 percent of U.S. primary and secondary education is provided by the public sector. In the United States, as in few other societies, there is a common acceptance of the idea—though too often a rejection of the burden the idea demands—that equity in education is a fundamental goal.

There are some societies—and China at times is one of them —which go further and contend that justice demands far more than equity, that those who work the hardest and have the least (the "prisoners of starvation," the "wretched of the earth") should have the most ("We have been naught, we shall be all," says the "Internationale") even if this interferes in the short run with capital accumulation and industrial development or other goals of the society.

Even those who would reject this view as applied to all of society's goods and services (whether on the basis of a long-term view of development or a short-term view of redistribution's impact on themselves and their privileged economic or social status) may be willing to accept it as applied to specific basic services such as health care. This willingness might be based on an acceptance of the need to redress past injustice, to compensate for current inequities in other areas, or simply to provide a safety valve to protect themselves against more far-reaching redistribution of wealth and power.

Health-care and medical-care services, in short, whatever else they do, in our view must—and can—be used to reduce inequities in the society. This goal is of course closely related to a more widely accepted goal for the health-care system, that of promotion and protection of health. It is our view that a society in which some people have and control a vast amount of the resources, while many others have and control very few of the resources, cannot achieve the goal of health for all its people, and may not be able to achieve the goal of health—in its broader sense of well-being—for any of them. But it should be clear that it is our view that the health-care and medical-care system must have equity and justice as a primary goal even if equity and justice do not contribute to "health" as conventionally defined.

There are several specific ways in which health-care services and medical-care services can contribute to the reduction of inequity and injustice. One method, commonly discussed in relation to health-care and medical-care services, is by guaranteeing equity, or more than equity, for those who are disadvantaged in their access to these services—the poor, the aged, the nonwhite, the sick and disabled. It is important to emphasize that equity (not to speak of more than equity) in health care and in medical care does not mean equality of access, does not mean "one person, one hospitalization" or even "one person, five doctor visits." Certain people, because of their illness or disability, their social or economic circumstances, or for other reasons, may require far more than their equal "share" of access to health care and medical care in order for equity to be achieved. Much has been made in recent years of the fact that for the first time those who are poor within our society have made a slightly greater number of doctor visits per patient per year than those who are affluent. But it must be noted at the same time that the poor have considerably more illness and disability than do the rich. There is little doubt that health-care and medical-care services are still inequitably distributed relative to need, and even if they were not, providing even greater service to the poor may help to even out other continuing inequities.

Another way in which the health-care and medical-care system can foster equity is through the jobs—the opportunities of serving others and of earning a livelihood—that it provides. These jobs, of course, may be distributed in such a way that they increase the inequity that exists in the society—which, as we shall see, is the current situation in the United States—or they may be used to decrease inequity. This goal, too, is inextricably bound up with the goal of maintaining and promoting health. It has been repeatedly stated that unemployment or lack of job satisfaction is in some fundamental sense unhealthy. Again, to make ourselves clear, we would argue that a goal of the health-care and medical-care system must be the reduction of inequity in employment even if that did not lead directly to better "health."

Overall, the health-care and medical-care system on which we spend over $150 billion per year and which constitutes 9 percent of our GNP can, through the ways in which it receives its income and the ways in which it disburses it, have a significant impact on equity. We will therefore examine, in the United States and in the other four countries which we are studying, the extent to which the health-care and medical-care systems lead toward, or away from, greater equity and justice.

2. We believe that the strengthening of individual, family and community life is a second fundamental goal of a society's health-care and medical-care system. Next to the guarantee of equity, in our view, societies have the responsibility of ensuring

each person the opportunity for a satisfying social existence. The health-care and medical-care system can, depending on how it is constructed by society, either contribute toward that goal or move society away from it. Health care and medical care can be superimposed upon a society so as to increase the individual's, family's and community's feelings of impotence and alienation and their disintegration, or, on the other hand, health care and medical care can be built into individual, family and community life in such a way as to strengthen them and utilize and maximize people's potential for mutual caring and healing.

This goal is also inextricably bound up with the notion of "health," since troubled individual, family or community life is surely an important factor in producing illness or disability. Yet again we would argue for this goal as itself one of the desired primary ends of a society's health-care and medical-care system, even if the goal did not itself contribute to better "health."

Overall, the health-care and medical-care system, as a major community institution, can, through its organization and function, have a significant impact on social life. We will examine each of the countries in an attempt to determine whether the health-care and medical-care system contributes to a sense of community and to personal feelings of strength and competence, or, rather, robs the individual and the collective of the ability for self-care and mutual aid.

3. We believe, of course, that the protection of health is also a fundamental goal of a health- and medical-care system. A society, in our view, has a clear obligation to protect its citizens, insofar as it is possible to do so, from environmental pollution, occupational hazards, infectious disease and other preventable causes of illness. A society is also responsible for providing for basic human needs, such as food, shelter, clothing and satisfying work, the absence of which inexorably leads to illness. The Preamble to the Constitution of the World Health Organization, which defines "health" broadly as "a state of complete physical, mental, and social well-being and not merely the absence of disease or infirmity," states also that "the enjoyment of the highest attainable standard of health is one of the

fundamental rights of every human being without distinction of race, religion, political belief, economic or social condition." It concludes: "Governments have a responsibility for the health of their peoples which can be fulfilled only by the provision of adequate health and social measures."

As we have noted, there are those who argue that medical care, and even health care as conventionally defined, make relatively little contribution to health compared to the contribution made by other societal conditions. Nonetheless we feel that the health-care and medical-care system can, if appropriately structured and combined with other societal efforts, make a significant contribution to health. We will examine each country in an attempt to assess how completely it has provided these services and the other "adequate health and social measures" which are essential to the "highest attainable standard of health."

4. Finally, we believe that care for the ill, or for the "worried well"—which includes appropriate diagnosis and appropriate advice, reassurance and, if necessary, treatment —is also an essential goal of a society's health-care and medical-care system. It is not by accident, however, that it has been placed last among our goals. We believe that medical care can be extremely dangerous as well as highly beneficial. It must therefore be controlled so as to do minimal harm—both in the sense of direct physical harm to the individual or the community and in the sense of creating increased dependency, inequity and fragmentation of family and community. Care must simultaneously include appropriate technical knowledge and skill; warm, humane, truly "caring" personnel; and the use of techniques culturally acceptable to the specific population.

We further believe that medical care must take an appropriate place in the health-care and medical-care system, not one of supremacy but rather alongside the promotion and protection of health and the guarantee of basic human needs. We will examine each of the societies to assess whether medical care, including an appropriate level of diagnosis and appropriate, humane treatment, is provided as one component of a broad, integrated system designed to promote a caring society.

There is danger, of course, in assigning to the health- and medical-care system too great a role within the society. It may be argued, quite rightly, that at least the first two and much of the third are goals which should be the responsibility of the larger society rather than specifically that of the health-care and medical-care system. It is possible that burdening "health care" —and especially burdening "medical care"—with the task of seeking all of these goals may make it that much harder to achieve the latter two highly specific goals of better health (in the narrow sense) and effective medical care.

And there is yet another danger. Assigning all four of these goals to the health-care and medical-care system in a society in which the system is controlled by professionals may give too much power to the professionals and thereby expropriate it from the community. Making promotion of equity, of community, or even of health, into "medical" goals, it is argued by some, may be itself counterproductive to the achievement of these goals. In short, there is a very narrow line between, on the one hand, making medical care and health care relevant to social problems and, on the other, making social problems into "medical" problems which become the province and property of professionals and of their technology.

While we are concerned mainly about the specific role of the health-care and medical-care system, we are concerned more broadly with achieving the fundamental social changes which will permit the emergence of a society in which justice, a sense of community, maximum attainable health, and competent, humane care can take place. We believe—another basic assumption—that such fundamental change is not only possible but inevitable. We believe that there are fundamental elements in the U.S. experience and in its belief system with which its social and health conditions—some of which we will document in this book—are in the most profound contradiction, and that out of that contradiction between just values and unjust practices will come the changes that we so urgently need.

On the one hand, we believe that health care and medical care can be a cutting edge—rather than one of the barriers—to change in other areas. Access to health care and medical care is widely and increasingly viewed in the United States as a right, one as fundamental as that of access to education or suffrage; it is hard to be against the idea of justice in health care and medical care. Health care and medical care in the United States are widely criticized, for performance as well as cost; it is hard to be against change, even fundamental change, in a relatively ineffective and extraordinarily expensive health-care and medical-care system. Good health care and, particularly, good medical care are widely seen as being of most potential benefit to those who are most disadvantaged—the very young, the very old, the sick and the disabled; it is hard to be against better care for those who are seen as among the most needy in the society. Finally those who dominate the health-care system, and particularly those who dominate the medical-care system and those who act as defenders of it, are widely seen as defending their own self-interests; it is hard to be against taking power and income away from those who are seen as profiting in wealth and power at the expense of those who are sick. For all of these reasons, the health-care system, we believe, is vulnerable to attempts at radical change, and the changes wrought can be used as models, as fulcrums, and as organizational bases for wider societal changes.

Health care and medical care are, of course, only one of the cutting edges leading to changes in the society at large. Those working in other areas can surely produce change which will also affect the larger society. It is the sum of these efforts drawing strength from each other, and their cumulative effect on the society as a whole, that will lead us toward the necessary societal change.

But what of the other side of the coin? Even if the health-care and medical-care system is indeed vulnerable to attempts at change, is a fundamental reconstruction of the system possible in the midst of this society? Can we hope to develop a just, caring, democratic and communal health-care and medical-care system in the midst of an unjust, technologized, deperson-alized, hierarchical and fragmented country? The answer, of course, is no. But we can come a great deal closer than we are now, and the very attempts to produce the change will them-selves have value, both for health care and medical care in the short run and for other areas in the society in the long run.

Furthermore, the redistribution of power and wealth which we believe is inevitable will not automatically bring the new society that we seek. Assumption of power by those who now have least power over the resources of society, while certainly a necessary condition for humane, caring and communal insti-tutions, is not itself a sufficient condition; much more ex-perimentation and much more experience with new models will be needed to forge social institutions which are rooted, at least in part, in American culture and will work in an American context, even after a democratic socialism—which we advocate —has been achieved. The models developed now—both the successes and the failures—can be used to influence the shape of institutions in the future.

We have stated some of the origins, the assumptions and the purposes that underlie this book. What is to be its method?

Part 1 is a selective catalog of some of the problems of health and of health care and medical care in the United States. Not all the important problems could be included; for example, little is said of promotion of mental health and of care for those with mental illness. On the other hand, since this is primarily a catalog of problems, some of the praise for the system has also been omitted. For many, particularly for those who feel them-selves to be well or for those who have the knowledge, the power or the money to bend the system to meet their needs, it seems to work well. However, since our primary goal is justice, these are not the people we are predominantly concerned with; in fact, as we point out in Part 3, they may very well be less satisfied—in the short run—with a more just system than with an unjust one.

Part 2, an exploration of alternatives as seen in other soci-eties, is in many ways the most difficult. Lack of detailed knowledge and lack of space to write a book on each country makes such analyses in some ways superficial. Our objective, however, is not a detailed analysis of health care in each country but the formulation of a set of relevant insights into how other societies have dealt with the issues of health care and medical care. Among the points we wish to make is that other countries have dealt with their problems in ways very different indeed from the ways in which we have dealt with them, and, perhaps even more important, in each country the health-care and the medical-care system is in some ways a result of that country's social, economic, political and cultural past. Great Britain with its National Health Service based around the general practitioner; Sweden with its mixture of public and private, centralized and decentralized health and medical care; the Soviet Union with its highly centralized, comprehensive system; and China with its emphasis on local participation—all represent efforts to evolve ways of providing health care which stem from the history and culture of each society and which attempt to meet some of the basic needs of the people.

In choosing these four we have slighted the insights to be gained from countries, such as Canada and Australia, with social conditions and health- and medical-care systems much closer to our own. The experiences of these countries have been discussed in depth elsewhere, however, and lessons from their experience have found their way into our recommendations. But we have chosen rather to emphasize countries with markedly different systems and with markedly different responses to problems we have in common, rather than countries with systems and responses basically similar to our own.

In Part 3 we attempt to present in brief the historical roots and current social background of health care and medical care in the United States. And in the final chapter we present what we view as the kind of system needed in the long run and our set of recommendations for short-run action which will bring us closer to the goals. The only thing that can be said with certainty is that our analysis of the roots and social context of the problems is incomplete and that the recommendations will not be followed in their entirety, and perhaps not at all. We also know from the experience of other countries that every change will bring new problems, even as it responds to ones we now have. But if the analysis and the recommendations contribute in some way—even a small one—to the formulation of appropriate responses and the march toward a more just, more caring, more democratic and more communal health-care and medical-care system, and a more just, communal, healthy and caring society, the effort will have been worthwhile.

In short, we view this book as a beginning, not a final word. We view it as an analysis in progress, not a final judgment. The greatest compliment the reader can give us is reasoned disagreement—part of a dialectic process out of which comes cogent analysis and effective action.

Part 1

Health Care and Medical Care in the United States

1

PROGRESS AND PROBLEMS: Power, Prestige and Profits

1. Despite unparalleled advances in medical technology—including powerful new methods for both diagnosis and treatment —and despite the skill and dedication of many health workers, the recognition grows, in every sector of our society, that something is seriously wrong with health care and medical care in the United States.

A crescendo of criticism engulfs the American health-care and medical-care system. Criticism is heard from every segment of society: from the healthy and the sick, from the high-rise in the megalopolis to the shack in the delta, from the board room to the loading dock, from the cattle rancher to the stoop laborer, from the rich, from the middle class and from the poor. Residents of the South Bronx and of the Lower East Side of New York City demonstrate to preserve old, dilapidated hospitals in their neighborhoods, fearing the loss of accessible health care, of long-familiar community institutions, and of jobs. Citizens of a small town in Kansas build a well-equipped office and a house in an effort to entice a doctor to settle among them, to no avail. The suburban mother can't reach her pediatrician to ask about the baby's fever, and ends up driving ten miles on an icy night to an emergency room.

Everywhere one hears the stories of the high costs, the impersonal care, the duplicated or missing lab tests and the long waits. And sometimes the stories have a sharper point: the death from a preventable illness or a preventable drug reaction;

the gallbladder surgery which was probably unnecessary or at least deferrable and which, in addition, did nothing to relieve the symptoms; the tales about doctors who are incompetent, rapacious, fraudulent or outright larcenous, and about the medical institutions that are more concerned with equipment than with people and so bureaucraticized that no one—patients, staff or the administrators themselves—is satisfied with them.

Indeed some of the most vehement voices of criticism are heard among those who provide medical care. The lowest-paid hospital workers strike to demand wage increases which at least meet the increases in the cost of living, or to protest massive layoffs. Interns and residents strike to protest long hours and inadequate facilities, for their own sake and, they say, for the benefit of their patients. Nurses strike for higher wages, a union shop and a louder voice in staffing decisions. And physicians strike to protest astronomic malpractice insurance rates. Doctors complain about their "bad press" and their feelings of being engulfed in increasing regulation and paper work. Nurses complain about the lack of appreciation of their work and inappropriate use of their professional skills. Medical-care administrators complain about undisciplined doctors and uncaring workers and inadequate funding for medical-care services. Medical workers complain about rigid and uncaring administrators and about the grossly inequitable distribution of the wealth which pours into the medical-care system.

The press and government add their voices. The Boston medical and nonmedical community is shocked to learn through their newspapers that a hospital technician has exposed an extraordinary, unnecessarily high death rate from heart surgery in a local community hospital in which relatively few such operations are performed; when the surgery is performed at hospitals in which this type of heart surgery is frequently done, a far lower death rate occurs. A U.S. Senate subcommittee charges "rampant fraud and abuse . . . among practitioners participating in the Medicaid program, matched by an equivalent degree of error and maladministration by government agencies." It further charges that from a quarter to a half of the $15 billion per year spent on Medicaid is being "wasted through fraud, poor quality of care, and the provision of services to ineligible persons." Almost simultaneously a U.S. House of Representatives subcommittee finds that failures of the Medicaid program in preventive medicine "caused unnecessary crippling, retardation, or even death of thousands of children."

What is particularly striking about the increasing criticism is that much of it comes from people in sectors of our society that find little fault with its basic structure, seek no fundamental redistribution of resources, no radical restructuring of relationships and no significant sharing of power. A 1970 issue of *Fortune* magazine, for example, was reprinted as a book whose introduction begins: "American medicine, the pride of the nation for many years, stands now on the brink of chaos."

In addition to articles on the rapidly increasing costs of medical care, *Fortune* addresses itself to issues of quality and competence. It quotes, for example, a Fellow of the American College of Surgeons and a leader of the New York State Medical Society, writing in the *New York State Journal of Medicine:* "Errors in judgment or technique concerning either the anesthesia or the surgery, or a combination of the two, contribute close to 50% of the mortality in the operating room." It cites the judgment, by an expert medical team from the Columbia University School of Public Health, that one-third of the hysterectomies performed on a sample of patients in hospitals in and around New York City had been "performed without any justification."

Fortune even recognizes the problems specifically faced by poor people: "Medical manpower and facilities are so maldistributed that large segments of the population, particularly the urban poor and those in rural areas, get virtually no care at all —even though their illnesses are most numerous and, in a medical sense, often easy to cure." And it summarizes: "Whether poor or not, most Americans are badly served by the obsolete, overstrained medical system that has grown up around them helter-skelter, without accommodating very well to changing technology, population, rising costs, or rising expectations."

At about the same time, the secretary of Health, Education

and Welfare in the Nixon administration declared that the differences between groups in the United States with regard to health status and health services had become "intolerable." He went further: "The indices of general improvement in health pale in importance when we look behind them and see that the poor and the nonwhites are doing far worse than whites and those with decent incomes. . . . When we look beyond our borders and compare ourselves with other nations any sense of accomplishment over our long-run gains in health status is mitigated by the fact that other advanced nations are doing better than we are. . . ."

In the years of the 1970s, since *Fortune* and the secretary of HEW made these statements, the criticisms have continued to grow both in scope and in intensity. The *New York Times*, for example, in early 1976 published a series of five front-page articles with headlines which read: "Unfit Doctors Create Worry in Profession," "Incompetent Surgery Is Found Not Isolated," "Thousands a Year Killed by Faulty Prescriptions," "Few Doctors Ever Report Colleagues' Incompetence," and "How Educated Patients Get Proper Health Care." That last, more hopeful headline was simultaneously balanced by another, as one turned to the continuation of the article on page ten: "Millions of X-rays Found Unneeded and Radiation Is Often Expensive."

The *Times* was clearly in step with the mood of the American people who seem to be growing ever more critical of medicine and ever less confident of its ability to meet their needs. The Harris poll, for example, indicates that the percentage of the public that has "a great deal of confidence in people in charge of running medicine" has declined from 73 percent in 1966 to 43 percent in 1977.

But there is a paradox here which the defenders of the current structure of the American medical-care system are quick to point out. The system which is being criticized from all sides is precisely the one that has been in the forefront of revolutionary changes in the technology of dealing with disease and disability since the turn of the century and at an increasing pace since World War II. Since Oliver Wendell Holmes told the

Massachusetts Medical Society in 1860, "I firmly believe that if the entire materia medica as now used could be sunk to the bottom of the sea, it would be all the better for mankind—and all the worse for the fishes," there have been dramatic discoveries of drugs and other methods of dealing with disease.

For example, during the 1920s hormones began to be available for patients who lacked enough of their own. During the 1930s and 1940s sulfa drugs and then penicillin and other antibiotics became available, helping the body to deal with infections it was unable to deal with on its own, or to speed recovery. Cortisone was introduced in the 1950s and facilitated the treatment of specific problems such as arthritis and asthma, and in the 1950s and 1960s potent new psychoactive agents were developed which had an extraordinarily beneficial effect in the care of psychotic patients.

As we shall discuss, these discoveries have also led, in an astonishing number of patients, to more illness; but it is undeniable that for untold millions they have been lifesaving and life-sustaining. Most of us today cannot imagine a world without antibiotics or insulin or cortisone or L-dopa or Thorazine.

Dramatic changes have also occurred in techniques of medical care other than medication. There have been, for example, spectacular advances in surgery: in the safety of anesthesia; in open-heart and other forms of cardiovascular surgery; in transplantation of tissues and organs; in treatment of severe burns; and in other operative procedures undreamed of a generation ago. Diagnostic systems have also changed markedly: The computed tomographic (CT) scanner, for example, using X-ray techniques in conjunction with a computer, can form a picture of internal body organs and provide clues to the diagnosis of disease without the necessity for diagnostic surgery or other methods that directly invade the body. Life-support systems have been markedly advanced, such as those for maintaining respiration and circulation until the body can again resume its own function.

Furthermore, the health status of the American people has vastly improved during this century. Life expectancy at birth in the United States in 1900 for white males was 47 years, for white females 49 years. In 1975 the comparable figures were 69 years and 77 years, a gain of 22 years for white males and 28 years for white females. Infant mortality for white babies in 1900 was approximately 70 deaths in the first year of life per 1000 live births (1 baby in 14 dying before its first birthday); for 1975 the estimated figure for white babies was 14.4 per 1000 (1 baby in 70). And the gains in life expectancy and infant survival for "nonwhite" people has been even greater, even though the levels are still significantly poorer than for "whites."

Not only have death rates decreased but many diseases—like smallpox, cholera, yellow fever, typhus fever, scarlet fever and polio—have completely or almost completely disappeared in the United States. The incidence of other once relatively common illnesses—like diphtheria and tetanus—have dropped to extremely low levels. Other illnesses—tuberculosis for example —are by no means conquered, but are markedly reduced in incidence.

Even some noninfectious illnesses now seem to be falling in incidence if one corrects for the increasing age of the population. By far the greatest single cause of death in the United States is heart disease, and of these deaths by far the largest number are due to coronary heart disease which killed almost 700,000 Americans in 1975. The death rate from coronary disease had been increasing steadily during most of this century, but current data suggest that the "age-adjusted" rate of deaths attributable to this cause plateaued between 1960 and 1967 and then began to fall. Indeed, the coronary death rate has apparently fallen by 13 percent in the five-year period between 1970 and 1975, a savings of about 15,000 lives per year.

Furthermore there is little doubt that health and medical workers in the United States are extremely well trained technically and that most of them work extraordinarily hard and with deep dedication. In contrast to the responses of a significant part of the public to questions regarding their confidence in medicine and their confidence in the medical profession in general, there appears to be a great deal of public confidence in the honesty and ethical standards of doctors as individuals, and in their own doctors in particular. Respondents to public opinion polls consistently place physicians second only to Supreme Court justices in their esteem, and although the absolute value of the percentage is surely less than the profession would like, and the overall results a sorry statement on the state of U.S. society, it is certainly significant that a 1976 Gallup poll showed physicians at the very top of a list of 11 occupations, with 55 percent of the respondents attributing "high" or "very high" ethical standards to them.

The technical knowledge and skill of most health workers, and the fact that the technology available to them for the medical care of their patients is—with the possible exception of Sweden's—the best in the world, explains why there must be very few Americans indeed who, stricken with a serious illness in a foreign land, would not prefer to be brought back to the United States for medical care.

Why then all the criticism? Why the myriad of recent books, articles, speeches, case histories and exposés? Where, in short, does health care and medical care in the United States really stand?

2. On the one hand, by commonly accepted measures, the people of the United States are less healthy than are the people of other comparably urbanized, industrialized and affluent countries, and, within the United States, some groups of people are by almost all measures demonstrably much less healthy than others.

By most comparable measures of health status the people of the United States are less healthy than are people in other technologically developed, wealthy countries. As we have noted, most of the factors influencing the health of a people lie outside what is conventionally defined as the responsibility of "medical care," and many of the most important ones lie outside the responsibility of conventionally defined "health care." These factors include individually inborn characteristics such as genetic inheritance and socially determined characteristics such as housing, nutrition and life-style. Nonetheless, since one of the generally accepted purposes of a health-care and medical-care system is promotion and protection of health, it may be relevant to begin by reviewing some comparative data on health and illness. A look at four commonly used criteria will suffice to make the point that health in the United States is poorer than it needs to be.

Death Rates and "Life Expectancy"

Death rates are the ones most often used for comparisons of health status between, and within, countries. The relative clarity of the definition of death (despite, in the case of a few dying people, a problem in defining the precise moment of "death") and the completeness of reporting of deaths (despite lapses in some of the poorer countries) make death rates much more reliable and comparable than rates of illness, disability, malnutrition or poor physical fitness, and infinitely more comparable than rates of positive good health. Death rates, in other words, may not be—and in some respects are probably not—the most important measures of the health status of a country, but they are by far the most reliable and comparable indicators.

Death rates in the United States at every age level except for the very oldest groups in the population are higher than in other comparably developed countries. Since the total death rate (technically known as the "crude death rate") of a country is more a reflection of the number of its older people than of the death rate at each age, "age-specific death rates" are used for comparison, as shown in Tables 1 and 2. Except for the oldest age groups, for 1973, the most recent year for which the World Health Organization has published comparable statistics, U.S. rates are consistently higher, for both males and females, than are those for England and Wales or Sweden. In all three countries the death rates for males are considerably higher than the rate for females; in the United States the difference is particularly pronounced.

TABLE 1

Age-Specific Death Rates for Males, 1973

(Deaths per 1000 population per year)

Age	Sweden	England & Wales	United States
Less than 1 yr.	10.8	18.9	19.9
1–4	0.5	0.8	0.9
5–14	0.3	0.4	0.5
15–24	1.0	1.0	1.9
25–34	1.2	1.0	2.1
35–44	2.4	2.3	3.8
45–54	5.5	7.2	9.2
55–64	14.3	20.4	22.1
65–74	38.2	51.5	47.3
75+	117.3	136.4	118.4
All Ages ("Crude death rate")	11.6	12.4	10.7

TABLE 2

Age-Specific Death Rates for Females, 1973

(Deaths per 1000 population per year)

Age	Sweden	England & Wales	United States
Less than 1 yr.	8.9	14.7	15.4
1–4	0.4	0.6	0.7
5–14	0.3	0.2	0.3
15–24	0.4	0.4	0.7
25–34	0.6	0.6	0.9
35–44	1.3	1.6	2.2
45–54	3.2	4.3	4.9
55–64	7.3	10.2	10.8
65–74	21.5	26.8	24.5
75+	88.6	101.0	86.4
All Ages ("Crude death rate")	9.4	11.5	8.1

From *World Health Statistics Annual, 1973–1976, Vol. 1, Vital Statistics and Causes of Death* (Geneva: World Health Organization, 1976).

If one examines the tables for each sex separately one finds, for example, that girls one to four years old in the United States had almost twice the chance of dying during 1973 that Swedish girls of the same age had. A 15-to-24-year-old in the United States, of either sex, had almost twice the chance of dying that an English young person had at the same age. A 25-to-34-year-old U.S. male had over twice the chance of dying that his English counterpart had, and a 45-to-54-year-old U.S. male had almost twice the chance of dying of one in Sweden. Only at the oldest ages were the "age-specific" rates in the United States at approximately the same levels as, or lower than, those in Sweden or England.

Similar differences may be found between areas within countries. In the United States startling differences occur between states, between areas within states, and even between contiguous sections of cities. Victor Fuchs has recently analyzed in detail the fact that, even though the states are contiguous, age-specific death rates in Nevada are considerably higher at all ages than in Utah. Fuchs's attribution of the differences almost exclusively to life-style and the conclusions he draws—which we would term "blaming the victim"—may be arguable, but the fact of the enormous differences in death rates of groups of people within a few miles of each other is not.

Age-specific death rates are often converted, by what can only be termed a statistical trick, into the widely reported indicator called "life expectancy," usually given as "life expectancy at birth," "life expectancy at age 40," or at some other specific age. The calculation of life expectancy, however, is based on an assumption that is clearly incorrect: that current age-specific death rates will remain constant for the remaining life of the group of people for whom the prediction is made. Therefore the calculation is flawed—and it may in fact be almost meaningless —if one is calculating life expectancy at birth or at some other young age.

An even more important problem, at least in the popular interpretation of widely publicized change in life expectancy, is the little-mentioned fact that in recent years almost all the improvement in "life expectancy at birth," the most commonly used figure, has been due to decreases in the death rate in the first year of life; "life expectancy" at later ages has improved little because the death rates at later ages have fallen little.

In short, "life expectancy" is an inadequate and often misleading shorthand for a series of age-specific death rates at every age. Since age-specific death rates for young and middle-aged Americans—particularly males—are considerably higher than in Sweden, Britain and other industralized countries, their "life expectancy" is consistently lower, and little information and less insight is gained by citing it. Nonetheless, since it is often cited, for the record let it be said here too that "life expectancy at birth," and at all ages up to age 65, is lower in the United States than in most comparably developed countries and that within the United States, although the gap has been narrowing somewhat in recent years, life expectancy at birth for nonwhite males is six years shorter than for white males, and five years shorter for nonwhite females than for white females. The differences in life expectancy at birth for males and females in selected countries are shown in Figure 1.

Far more important than "life expectancy" in making comparisons are more specific, and therefore more comparable, death rates. It is for this reason that the most widely internationally compared death rate is the infant mortality rate—the number of live-born babies dying in their first year of life per 1000 live births. The U.S. infant mortality rate, despite recent declines, remains almost double that of the country with the lowest rate (Sweden) and 50 percent higher than the rates in countries like the Netherlands, Japan and Switzerland.

It has often been noted—usually by apologists for the relatively high rates in the United States—that there are problems with comparisons of infant mortality among different countries. Indeed there are. It is not clear, for example, that all countries use similar criteria in distinguishing between babies born alive and then dying shortly after birth, and babies already dead at birth. Most countries, including the U.S., attempt to include in the statistics all babies alive at the time of birth. France and

FIGURE 1

Life Expectancy at Birth for Selected Countries in the Early 1970s

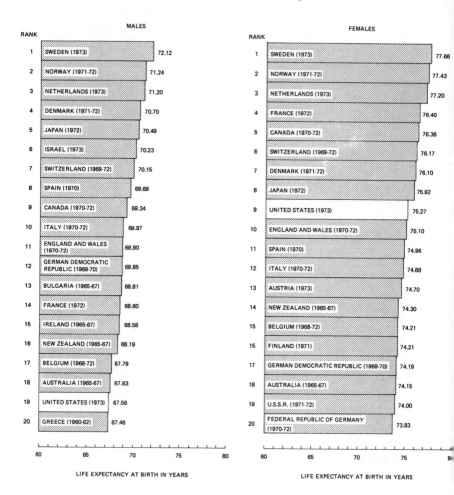

MALES

RANK		
1	SWEDEN (1973)	72.12
2	NORWAY (1971-72)	71.24
3	NETHERLANDS (1973)	71.20
4	DENMARK (1971-72)	70.70
5	JAPAN (1972)	70.49
6	ISRAEL (1973)	70.23
7	SWITZERLAND (1969-72)	70.15
8	SPAIN (1970)	69.69
9	CANADA (1970-72)	69.34
10	ITALY (1970-72)	68.97
11	ENGLAND AND WALES (1970-72)	68.90
12	GERMAN DEMOCRATIC REPUBLIC (1969-70)	68.85
13	BULGARIA (1965-67)	68.81
14	FRANCE (1972)	68.60
15	IRELAND (1965-67)	68.58
16	NEW ZEALAND (1965-67)	68.19
17	BELGIUM (1968-72)	67.79
18	AUSTRALIA (1965-67)	67.63
19	UNITED STATES (1973)	67.56
20	GREECE (1960-62)	67.46

60 65 70 75 80

LIFE EXPECTANCY AT BIRTH IN YEARS

FEMALES

RANK		
1	SWEDEN (1973)	77.66
2	NORWAY (1971-72)	77.43
3	NETHERLANDS (1973)	77.20
4	FRANCE (1972)	76.40
5	CANADA (1970-72)	76.36
6	SWITZERLAND (1969-72)	76.17
7	DENMARK (1971-72)	76.10
8	JAPAN (1972)	75.92
9	UNITED STATES (1973)	75.27
10	ENGLAND AND WALES (1970-72)	75.10
11	SPAIN (1970)	74.96
12	ITALY (1970-72)	74.88
13	AUSTRIA (1973)	74.70
14	NEW ZEALAND (1965-67)	74.30
15	BELGIUM (1968-72)	74.21
15	FINLAND (1971)	74.21
17	GERMAN DEMOCRATIC REPUBLIC (1969-70)	74.19
18	AUSTRALIA (1965-67)	74.15
19	U.S.S.R. (1971-72)	74.00
20	FEDERAL REPUBLIC OF GERMANY (1970-72)	73.83

60 65 70 75 80

LIFE EXPECTANCY AT BIRTH IN YEARS

Prepared by the National Center for Health Statistics, from data in the *United Nations Demographic Yearbook 1974,* for testimony before the U.S. Senate Health Subcommittee on March 31, 1977. Note that the scales begin with a life expectancy of 60 rather than 0 years; the figure therefore shows *absolute* differences rather than *relative* differences in life expectancy between countries.

Spain, however, beginning in 1973, have excluded live-born infants dying before registration of birth from both the live-birth data and the infant-death data. The USSR excludes infants of less than 28 weeks gestation, less than 1000 grams (two pounds) in weight and less than 35 centimeters (14 inches) in length who die within seven days of birth.

These problems of comparison are relatively small, however, compared with the overall rates and with the differences in rates among countries. Even if one counts only countries of over one million population and with "complete" counts of live births and infant deaths as defined by the United Nations, 14 countries, as shown in Figure 2, some of them—such as East Germany or Finland—considerably less affluent than the United States, had lower infant mortality rates than ours in the most recent year for which comparable data are available.

Even if one limits the comparison to white babies, the United States was no better than the tenth among the countries of the world in infant mortality in 1974. More alarming, the United States, which 25 years ago ranked much higher among the world's countries, has steadily lost its position—even as its infant mortality rate has fallen—as other countries reduced their infant mortality rates at a far faster rate. There have been further declines in the U.S. infant mortality rate in the past few years, and the U.S. position relative to other countries may now be beginning to improve —although that is not yet clear—but that still cannot make up for the thousands of infant deaths that might have been prevented over the past two decades.

Even more disturbing than the international differences are the differences in death rates between groups within the United States. Since the possible underlying causes of these differences are closely related to each other, the differences are difficult to assign to single causes. Poverty is certainly a critical component. Not by accident, however, the wealth, income, education, job classification—or other direct measures of social class— during the life of the deceased is not usually recorded on death

FIGURE 2

Infant Mortality Rates for Selected Countries in the Early 1970s

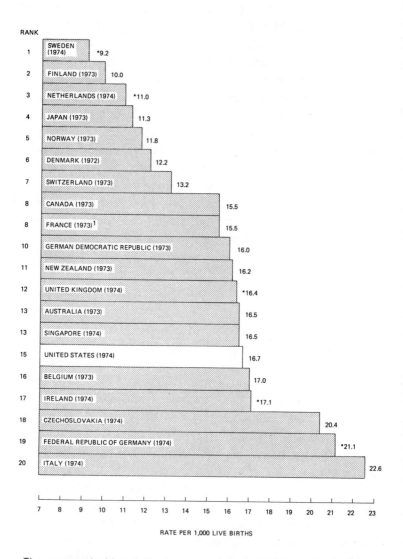

The rates marked by an (*) were provisional. The 1974 rate of 12.1 for France was not used because it includes live-born infants dying before registration of birth. Note that the scale begins with a rate of 7 rather than a rate of 0; the figure therefore shows *absolute* differences rather than *relative* differences in rate between countries. SOURCE: See Figure 1.

certificates in the United States. "Race" and residence address at the time of death are recorded, though, and these are the data used in most analyses.

Analyzed by "race," the 1974 infant mortality rate among "white" infants in the United States was 14.8 deaths in the first year of life per 1000 live births; among "nonwhite" infants it was 24.9 deaths per 1000 births, almost twice the rate. Analyzed geographically, U.S. infant mortality ranged from a low of 11.3 (in a "health service area" in Massachusetts) to a high of 27.1 (in an area in South Carolina), the highest rate more than double the lowest.

Special studies are needed to examine the effects of poverty directly. One such study, performed by the U.S. National Center for Health Statistics of infant mortality in poverty and non-poverty areas of 19 large cities of the United States from 1969 to 1971, showed that "whites" living in poverty areas had an infant mortality rate almost 50 percent higher than that of "whites" living in nonpoverty areas, and that "blacks," while having a higher rate than the "whites" in either type of area, also have a far higher infant mortality rate in poor areas than in nonpoor areas. In short, all three factors—poverty, "race" and residence—seem associated with greater numbers of dead babies.

If one looks specifically at those infant deaths which would appear to be preventable, the differences are even more disturbing. A small number of infant deaths seem un-preventable; some babies are born with such severe physical defects that their lives can't—and, some would say, shouldn't—be saved. If we assume that the infant mortality rate in Sweden, the country with the lowest rate (11 deaths per 1000 births), was the minimum one achievable in 1969–71 with the then current state of knowledge of how to care for pregnant women and their babies, then the "excess" deaths among babies born in nonpoor areas in the United States in those years was 6 per 1000 births and the "excess" deaths among babies born in poor areas was 13 per 1000 births. In other words, the probably preventable deaths in poor areas were over 100 percent higher than those in the nonpoor areas rather than "merely" 50 percent higher. Analyzed the same way, the "excess" deaths among "non-white" infants born in 1974 (15.7 per 1000) was almost three times as great as the "excess" deaths among "white" infants (5.6 per 1000). Furthermore, while deaths among infants after one month of age ("postneonatal infant deaths") are especially susceptible to preventive actions, during 1969–73 the rates for these deaths among health-service areas in the United States varied from a high of 13.6 per 1000 live births (in Arizona) to 2.9 per 1000 (in Connecticut), a ratio of over four to one.

There is, as we have noted, considerable controversy over the international comparability of infant mortality rates. But there is relatively little controversy over the comparability of maternal mortality rates—the number of mothers dying due to complications of childbirth per 100,000 live births.

The United States in 1950 had the lowest maternal mortality rate in the world (70 deaths per 100,000 births). But although the maternal mortality rate has fallen even lower since 1950, it has fallen considerably faster in many other countries; as shown in Table 3, the percent decrease in maternal mortality from 1960 to 1971 was lower for the United States than for any of the other countries listed. As a result, by 1971 at least nine other countries had lower maternal mortality rates than did the United States. The 1971 U.S. rate (20 deaths per 100,000 births) was two and a half times that of Sweden (8 per 100,000) and almost four times that of Denmark (5.3 per 100,000). In other words, in proportion to the number of births, four women died as a result of pregnancy and birth in the United States for every one who died of similar causes in Denmark. There has been a further reduction of maternal mortality in the United States since 1971—in part because of liberalized abortion laws—but our rates remain higher than those of other industrialized countries.

TABLE 3

Maternal Mortality in Selected Countries, 1960–1971

(Deaths due to childbirth per 100,000 live births)

1960		1971		Percent Decrease 1960–1971
Australia	52.5	Australia	18.5	65
Belgium	40.7	Belgium	20.4 (1970)	50
Canada	44.9	Canada	18.3	59
Denmark	30.2	Denmark	5.3	82
England and Wales	39.5	England and Wales	16.9	57
Finland	71.8	Finland	8.1	89
Japan	130.6	Japan	45.2	65
Netherlands	39.4	Netherlands	12.1	69
Norway	42.0	Norway	19.6	53
Sweden	37.2	Sweden	7.9	79
Switzerland	57.2	Switzerland	27.0	53
U.S.A	37.1	U.S.A	20.5	45

From Robert Maxwell, *Health Care: The Growing Dilemma* (New York: McKinsey & Co., 1975), Table 5, drawn from the *World Health Statistics Reports* published regularly by the World Health Organization, Geneva.

Preventable deaths, of course, occur at ages other than infancy and at times other than childbirth. Among the problems in international comparisons of such deaths is that death rates due to specific illness vary considerably from country to country and, perhaps even more important, the standards of reporting by physicians of cause of death on death certificates vary enormously from country to country.

Nevertheless, it appears, for example, that U.S. men aged 35–44 appear to be almost three times as likely to die of cardiovascular disease or of respiratory diseases as Swedish men of the same age. Death rates in this age group from cancer or from accidents, poisoning or violence are, on the other hand, only slightly greater in the United States. In the other direction, although reporting may be particularly unreliable for this cause of death, the Swedish rate for suicide (for the entire population) is almost double that of the United States.

A recent U.S. study identified some 70 medical conditions that can and should, in the present state of knowledge, be successfully prevented or managed. Yet in 1974 there were, exclusive of infant deaths, over 200,000 deaths from these 70 conditions, which include several different types of cancer, respiratory diseases and accidents.

Lung cancer, for example, is the most common type of cancer among men and the fastest rising type of cancer among women. It has been reliably estimated that some 90 percent of lung cancer could be prevented by abstinence from cigarette smoking. The U.S. Department of Health, Education and Welfare unequivocally states that "cigarette smoking remains the largest single preventable cause of illness and early death" in the United States. Yet attempts to induce people to give up cigarette smoking or, better still, to make sure they never start smoking are pitifully inadequate compared to the resources that are spent on cigarette advertising.

The rate of deaths from accidents, suicides and homicides in the United States is almost double that of the United Kingdom. Automobile accidents are the leading cause of death among Americans from age 1 through 38. There are some 50,000 deaths (and two million injuries) caused by the automobile each year, more than the number of deaths among U.S. troops in the entire 15 years of our involvement in Indochina. Other countries, such as Sweden, have materially reduced the deaths (and injuries) from automobiles by making the use of seat belts mandatory and by imposing heavy penalties—including imprisonment—on drivers with even a small amount of alcohol in their bloodstreams.

In 1975 almost 12,000 people also died as a result of fires, the highest fire-death rate of all industrialized nations in the world.

In short, there is good evidence that a significant number of people in the United States, particularly men, die at an earlier age than the experience of other countries or the experience of other groups within the United States suggests they need to; and that those who are poor, who are "nonwhite," or who live in certain areas of the country are more likely to die an early

—and probably preventable—death than are their fellow citizens.

Illness Rates

Rates of illness are far harder to compare cross-nationally than deaths. Not only do definitions of what constitutes, for example, a "common cold" or a "mild stroke" differ, but capabilities of reporting vary widely from country to country. Many U.S. doctors do not bother to report even those illnesses they are required by law to report.

While some argument may be made for maintenance of confidentiality in the case of socially stigmatized illnesses such as venereal disease (although even here the general feeling among public health workers, as contrasted with the feeling of many practicing physicians, is that the positives which come out of case-finding, treatment and prevention outweigh the negatives of disclosure), there would appear to be no excuse whatever for not reporting cases of a preventable and "socially acceptable" disease such as measles. Yet the U.S. Center for Disease Control estimates that only 10 percent of the measles cases in the United States are reported; a study in New York State showed that fewer than 5 percent of general practitioners and pediatricians reported any measles cases at all in 1971, a year of relatively high incidence of measles.

Even worse, there are large differences in reporting among areas within the United States. Thus, for the incidence of illness —as, to a lesser extent, for the exact causes of deaths—there is not even adequate information on which to base precise statements of health status.

Nonetheless, it is clear that preventable illnesses such as measles still unnecessarily strike down our children, leading in some cases of measles to encephalitis or other complications, to permanent disability or even death. A vaccine to prevent measles has been available since 1963, and there is no need for another child ever again to have measles, yet over one-third of American children one to four years of age have not been immunized against the disease. In the slums of our cities the rate of immunization is unknown but is certainly even lower than the overall rate; in parts of the South Bronx well over 50 percent of the preschool children, perhaps as many as three-fourths of them, are unprotected.

It is no surprise that those who are poor have a far greater chance of becoming sick—particularly a greater chance of becoming sick from preventable illness—than those who are not. Recent outbreaks of measles in the United States have concentrated among the poor and the nonwhite: In outbreaks in Los Angeles, Houston, Dallas and Little Rock, the reported rates among black children were three to *fifty* times as high as the rates among white children.

Rates of tuberculosis and venereal disease—in fact, rates of almost all forms of communicable disease and of injury and death due to accidents and violence—are far higher in poor areas than in affluent ones. The study by the National Center for Health Statistics of poverty and nonpoverty areas of 19 large U.S. cities, which we cited in connection with infant mortality, showed that "whites" living in poverty areas have a far higher rate of these illnesses than do "whites" living in nonpoverty areas, and that "nonwhite" people living in poverty areas have similarly higher rates than "nonwhite" people living outside such areas.

Furthermore, many forms of preventable illness in the United States are associated with medical care itself. For example, it is estimated that 20,000 to 30,000 patients receiving blood transfusions in the United States contract hepatitis. As Richard Titmuss pointed out in *The Gift Relationship,* in countries where blood donations are truly voluntary rather than paid for in some way, there is far less incentive for a donor to lie about a history of hepatitis before giving blood. As we shall explore later in this chapter, excessive health risks in the United States are also associated with high rates of use of medications, particularly antibiotics, and with high rates of elective surgery, such as hysterectomies and tonsillectomies.

In short, although the evidence is less precise and reliable than that for deaths, rates of certain preventable illnesses seem to be high in the United States, probably higher than in other industrialized countries and certainly far higher among the poor and the nonwhite than among the affluent.

Disability Rates

It is harder still to compare rates of disability between or within countries, since definitions and reporting of disability vary even more widely than they do for acute illnesses. One of the few well-controlled international comparative studies of disability was that performed in 1968–69 by the World Health Organization International Collaborative Study of Medical Care Utilization in twelve study areas in seven countries: four areas in Canada, two in the United States, two in Yugoslavia, and one each in Argentina, Finland, Poland and the United Kingdom. These study areas were chosen on the basis of the availability of local investigators with an interest in the study and may not be typical of the countries in which they are located; the two U.S. study areas, for example, were a five-county region in northwestern Vermont, and the city of Baltimore and its five surrounding counties. Representative samples of people in the study areas were interviewed in their homes using standardized questionnaires.

A person was defined as "healthy" if he or she did not report any of five indicators of ill health: (1) "social dysfunction" (days spent in bed or in restricted activity because of illness); (2) "perceived morbidity" (illness reported by the respondent); (3) specific symptoms (for example, chest pain or shortness of breath); (4) "perceived dental morbidity"; and (5) "perceived visual morbidity." A person was defined as "functionally healthy" if he had evidence of a mild level of illness or symptoms, or if he had recently visited a physician but did not report any recent days in bed or days of restricted activity.

The "healthy" people in the 12 study areas, mostly children

and young adults, ranged from 120 to 164 per 1000. The "functionally healthy" ranged from 210 to 286 per 1000. Overall, about 4 out of every 10 people were not impaired by illness in their functioning.

Taken together, two points emerge. First is the remarkable consistency of these data across a wide range of cultures and social conditions; it is evidence that cross-national comparisons of health- and medical-care services may have a comparable base of "health" in the population. The second is the extremely large percentage of the population (6 out of 10) who report disability of one sort or another.

In terms of specific measures of disability, the people of Baltimore and northwestern Vermont came out rather well, particularly compared to respondents in Poland and Yugoslavia. For example, the number of "sick days"—days when the respondent was in bed or was restricted in his activity because of illness over the two weeks prior to the interview—was about 600 days per 1000 people in the area of Vermont studied and about 800 days per 1000 people in the area of Maryland. This may be compared with about 1700 days per 1000 in the Polish city and 1500 and 1200 days per 1000 in the two Yugoslavian cities.

One of the leaders of the study comments that these differences may in part "reflect cultural differences in the manifestation of sickness rather than differences in illness as determined clinically." On the other hand, the numbers of sick days in the U.S. study areas are not very different from those in the study areas in Canada or England, Vermont's figure being close to those of the Canadian areas and Baltimore's being close to that of Liverpool.

Even a rate which is fairly easy to define and which would appear to be related to illness and "disability," such as days lost from work, may be much more related to social factors than to levels of comparable illness or disability. A study in the 1950s showed that the United States and Canada had extremely low rates of "sick absence" from work compared, for example, to the Federal Republic of Germany (West Germany).

Before the United States congratulates itself on how healthy its work force was, however, it should be noted that the unemployment rate in the United States and Canada was far higher, even then, than in West Germany. The low sick-absence rate may be more related to fear of being replaced by someone with less absenteeism or, probably a more important factor, that those who are often absent are less likely to be employed, than to "truly" lower levels of illness or disability among people of working age in the United States.

Since international differences in disability are extremely difficult to determine or to interpret, it appears far more important to consider differences between groups within the United States.

Surveys using standard definitions, done regularly by the U.S. Public Health Service, consistently show that the poor have much more chronic illness and disability than do those who are not poor. While it is not clear to what extent one is cause and the other is effect, people aged 17–44 with family incomes under $5000 in the early 1970s had a 30 percent higher prevalence rate of chronic conditions such as arthritis and heart conditions, and a 50 percent higher rate of diabetes, hypertension, hearing impairments and vision impairments than do those with incomes higher than $15,000.

The poor in this age group also lose 50 percent more days from work each year and have 100 percent more (twice as many) days of restricted activity and days of bed disability than do the wealthy; while 2.5 percent (one in every 40) of those in this age group with low incomes had limitation of mobility (defined as "confined to the house, needs help in getting around, or had trouble getting around alone"), only 0.4 percent (1 in every 250) of those in the high-income category had similar limitations.

Similar differences occur in other age groups and will be discussed later in this chapter. In short, although the extent to which poverty causes illness and illness causes poverty is still debated, what is unquestionable is that the poor in the United States are much sicker and more disabled than are the wealthy.

Malnutrition and Poor Physical Fitness

The rates of less clearly definable characteristics of ill health are hardest of all to measure, but may in the long run be the most important. Some 20 percent of people in the United States —particularly among the poor and the elderly—have inadequate amounts or types of food to meet their bodily needs. It has been estimated that 26 million Americans cannot afford an adequate diet and that, in 1973, when the report was prepared, almost half of them received no help whatever from any federal food program.

More subtle but in some ways even more telling, the average height of ten-year-old children of families with incomes below poverty level is significantly less than that of the ten-year-olds of families with incomes above poverty level. While American children have, on the average, been growing taller over the past century, the average height for poor children lags behind that for nonpoor children by more than a generation. This is not due to a difference in height associated with race, for the average height of black children is slightly more than that of white children of the same income level. Sweden in comparison has in recent years managed to eliminate growth differences between social classes, so far as is known the first country in the world to do so.

Furthermore, study after study has demonstrated the poor physical fitness of the American people. It was found in the early 1960s that one-third of all young men in the United States failed to meet the standards for induction into the armed forces, about one-half of these because of disease and disability and about one-half through inability to qualify on the mental test. The president's Task Force on Manpower Conservation found that "although many persons are disqualified for defects that probably could not be avoided in the present state of knowledge, the majority appear to be victims of inadequate education and insufficient health services."

Summary

Despite the highly publicized drop in U.S. death rates—and specifically in infant mortality rates—and despite the dramatic and even more highly publicized improvements in medical technology in recent years, the health status of the American people on the whole remains unsatisfactory. This is true whether viewed in absolute numbers of people dying, sick, disabled or unfit, compared by commonly accepted measures of illness in other affluent countries, or measured internally by comparing the health of some groups in the population with the health of others.

3. On the other hand, the U.S. health- and medical-care system is the most expensive one in the world, its cost is growing, profits and incomes can be enormous, and insurance coverage for the cost of care for individuals and families is generally inadequate.

The overall cost of health care and medical care in the United States (our "national health expenditures") for the year ending in June 1976 was $139 billion dollars, a mean of $638 for every man, woman and child in the United States. This represents by far the greatest expenditure for health and medical services of any country on the face of the earth. Even when measured as a fraction of this country's Gross National Product—the total of the goods and services the country produces—the magnitude of U.S. health expenditures is impressive: 8.6 percent of the U.S. GNP is now spent on health and medical care. Only Sweden, which, it is estimated, now also spends approximately 8 percent of its GNP on health, comes close. Great Britain, conversely, spends only about 5.5 percent of its GNP (which furthermore is far smaller per capita than either that of the United States or Sweden) for health services. Data for the USSR are difficult to compare, but it appears that approximately 6 percent of the "national budget" is devoted to health services.

Of equal, if not greater, significance than the current level of U.S. health expenditures is their rate of increase. In terms of total number of dollars spent, the increase in 25 years is staggering, from $12 billion in 1950 to almost $120 billion in 1975, the tenfold increase shown in Figure 3. The figure also shows that in these 25 years the "public" share (the portion supported by taxes or by social security levy funds) increased from 25 percent to 40 percent of the total.

More meaningful comparisons of total expenditure, however, require that the dollars expended must be adjusted to take into account the increase in the U.S. population, the inflation, and the expansion of the entire economy (a measure of the rise in our overall standard of living) during the quarter-century. The population of the United States increased from 150 million to 215 million in the past 25 years, an increase of over 40 percent. The per capita increase in health expenditures, as shown in Figure 4, was therefore about sevenfold—from about $80 per capita in 1950 to about $550 per capita in 1975.

Correction for the decreasing value of the dollar and for the general expansion in the economy during the same period is more difficult. One commonly used method is to show health expenditures as a fraction of the total U.S. GNP, as in Figure 5. The rise since 1950, not nearly as dramatic as in uncorrected total dollars, is about twofold—from 4.6 percent of the GNP in 1950 to 8.3 percent in 1975. This change represents, for most comparative purposes, a better measure of the increase in use of health services and the change in their nature and cost during the period. In the two years after price controls on the health care industry were lifted in 1974, national health expenditures rose by 31 percent compared to an 18 percent increase in the GNP, rising to their current share of almost 9 percent of GNP.

The change in the nature and use of services—particularly the introduction and expansion of the use of costly ones—are more dramatic when one looks at care for specific illnesses and the use of specific techniques. The number of laboratory tests for the average patient with a perforated appendix, for example, increased sixfold from 1951 to 1971. The number of diagnostic

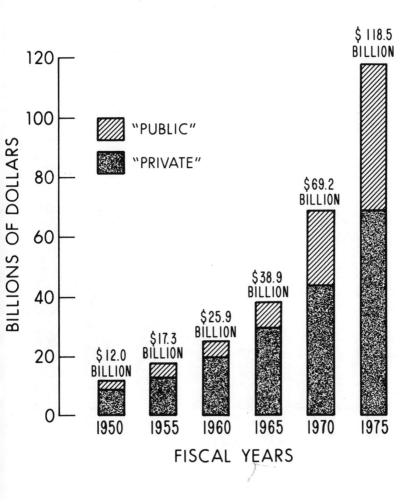

FIGURE 3

National Health Expenditures in the United States, 1950–1975

Prepared by the authors from data published by the Office of Research and Statistics of the Social Security Administration.

FIGURE 4

National Health Expenditures per Capita in the United States, 1950–1975

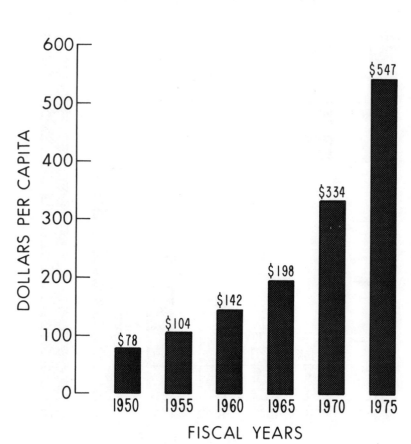

Prepared by the authors from data published by the Office of Research and Statistics of the Social Security Administration.

FIGURE 5

National Health Expenditures in the United States as a
Percentage of the Gross National Product, 1950–1975

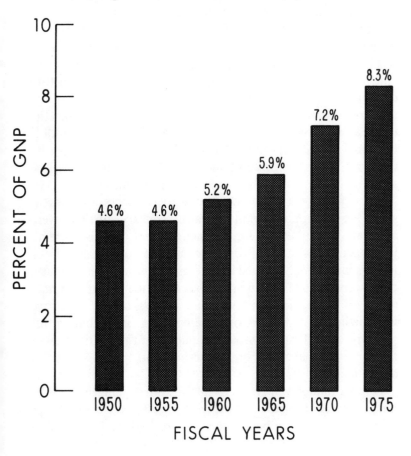

Prepared by the authors from data published by the Office of Research and
Statistics of the Social Security Administration.

X rays taken for a patient with cancer of the breast increased threefold, and the number of radiotherapy treatments for the patient with breast cancer increased sixfold. The number of electrocardiograms taken on a patient with myocardial infarction doubled from 1964 to 1971 alone. Even for maternity care the number of lab tests almost trebled from 1951 to 1971.

The number and types of new forms of diagnostic equipment and new forms of treatment boggle the mind. Hemodialysis (use of "artificial kidneys") and new forms of surgery are some of the most dramatic and well publicized. Yet these are only the tip of an iceberg of expensive technological change. Overall it is estimated that if the current pattern of increase continues, by the early 1980s over $200 billion ($1000 per person) will be spent annually on health care in the United States.

But high costs in and of themselves are not necessarily unreasonable or insupportable in a wealthy country—if there were adequate value received for the money spent, if there were no less expensive way to get the same or greater value, and if, for what is increasingly viewed as a necessity rather than a luxury, there were ways of making sure that everyone had appropriate access to the services without financial catastrophe. Later we will further explore some of these complex issues, but in this section we will limit ourselves to analysis of the distribution of the burden for paying for health services, and of the distribution of the income.

Approximately 90 percent of total health expenditures in the United States are spent on "personal" health services and supplies—items of direct benefit to the individual, such as hospital care, physicians' services and drugs. Only about 10 percent of total health expenditures are spent in "nonpersonal" areas, such as environmental and occupational health, disease detection and control, medical research, medical education, and construction of medical facilities. Public funds (from taxes and social security payments) pay almost all the cost of the "nonpersonal" services, but also pay an increasing portion of the costs of personal medical care as well.

The distribution of sources for personal health care and medical care expenditures from 1929 to 1975 is shown in Figure 6. Not only has the percentage covered by public funds doubled since 1950, but the percentage covered by private health insurance has almost tripled. Therefore, overall, the percentage of personal health care expenditures covered by direct payments has halved, from two-thirds of the expenditures to one-third of the expenditures.

Thus an increasing share of even the so-called private funds are really communally controlled funds—funds collected and pooled by insurance companies, who, together with government, are the "third-party payers" through which the vast bulk of the the money paid into the health-care and medical-care system flows. The insurance funds, while technically "private," are largely under "communal" rather than "individual" control.

In short, only a smaller and smaller proportion of the funding for health care is met by truly "private" individual payments at the time of service, and over two-thirds of the costs are paid by pooled communal funds of one type or another. The market mechanism in medicine is largely a myth. Individual choice in payment for care—and often in the source of care—is largely nonexistent. Increasingly, communities and the society as a whole, rather than individuals, have the power to determine how much of their resources they are willing to allocate to health and medical care, and to what purposes they want these resources used.

Looked at another way, the percentage of personal income spent on personal medical care has risen sharply over the last 25 years. In 1952, out of a total of $250 billion personal income for all people in the United States, a total of $14 billion (5.1 percent) was paid for personal medical care. By 1962 personal income in the United States had almost doubled, to $443 billion, but personal medical expenditures had more than doubled, to $29 billion or 6.5 percent of income. By 1972 the respective figures were $936 billion (somewhat more than double that of 1962) and $80 billion (almost triple) or 8.5 percent of income spent on personal medical care. In 1952 an American worker

FIGURE 6

Sources of Funds for Personal Health Care
Expenditures in the United States, 1929–1975

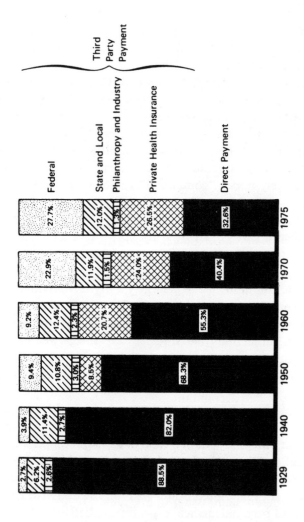

Prepared by the Office of Research and Statistics of the Social Security Administration. The years refer to fiscal years.

on the average spent about two and a half weeks' pay a year on personal medical services; by 1972 he or she spent about one month's pay a year.

It would be bad enough if this burden were equitably distributed among U.S. families. Of course it is not. A study performed by the Congressional Budget Office estimated that seven million families would have out-of-pocket medical expenditures exceeding 15 percent of their gross income during fiscal year 1978. These families would spend two months' pay or more a year for medical care.

A large, constant and predictable drain on the budget of low-income families, or even middle-income families, for medical care is problem enough, but the most extreme impact of the personal medical-care cost problem is felt by the family involved in the care of a catastrophic illness of one of its members. Stories of families bankrupted by, or chained for years to payment for, a complex sequence of care of even a single prolonged episode of hospitalization are well known. One example of such a catastrophe will suffice; it is the one with which Daniel Schorr begins his book *Don't Get Sick in America,* based on a 1971 "CBS Reports" program.

Johan van der Sande had emigrated to the United States from the Netherlands in 1957 at the age of 33, and by 1965, as van der Sande said, he felt like "a real Californian," with a family that included two adopted children, a $1000-a-month job as a certified public accountant, and a home, complete with mortgage. But in 1966 he began having a series of disabling symptoms and was found to have high blood pressure. He was treated with various medications, but the disability increased and he was forced to change jobs several times.

By 1969 van der Sande's kidneys had failed to such an extent that he required admission to Mt. Sinai Medical Center in Los Angeles for treatment which included hemodialysis (treatment with an artificial kidney machine). His bills, as he left the hospital, added up to $22,000. Approximately $20,000 was covered by his excellent Blue Cross policy, but the home dialysis unit that he needed required a first-year investment of

$25,000 and a continuing expenditure of $5000 per year. A group of friends formed a "van der Sande Kidney Fund," but after an initial burst, contributions began to taper off.

At this point van der Sande's family in Holland suggested that, since he had never adopted American citizenship, he could return to his home in the Netherlands. There, under the National Health Insurance Plan, for a premium of $24 a month he would receive full coverage of hospital, doctors and drug bills—and an artificial kidney machine at no additional charge to him.

"In America," commented van der Sande in 1971, back again at his home in Nymegen where he was interviewed by CBS correspondent Morley Safer, "even if I could get help, I would have to be dependent on charity. I would have to hold out my hand and say, 'Will you help me please?' People here," he continued, "were amazed at what friends did for me in California. But in Holland that would not be necessary. . . . In Holland you have a right. The taxpayers pay into a fund, and everybody has a right to be taken care of. . . . If I were a healthy person I would go back to America tomorrow. But, being sick, I don't dare go back to America. I feel that America is a good place to live if you're healthy. But don't get sick in America!"

In an effort to prevent financial disaster should they be faced with overwhelming personal medical-care costs, most people in the United States carry some form of health insurance. But, reflective of the costs of medical care and particularly of the cost of hospital care, premium rates for "nonprofit" health insurance (policies written by companies such as Blue Cross and Blue Shield in each state) and for "commercial" health insurance (such as those written by many different insurance companies) have also risen enormously in recent years. When written into labor contracts as fringe benefits, as they now often are, they take away from wage increases or from other forms of benefits. The automobile industry, for example, paid from 20 to 34 percent more for collectively bargained health insurance in 1975 than they had paid for the same insurance in 1974; in contrast, wages rose only 7 to 9 percent during the same period.

Furthermore, the only types of private health insurance that are really widespread in the United States are coverage for hospitalization and for surgical services; and even these are held by only slightly more than three-fourths of people under age 65, leaving some 40 million people under age 65 wholly unprotected by any form of private health insurance. Indeed, the percentage of people under age 65 covered by hospital insurance has remained static at about 75 percent over the past 10 years. Furthermore, while 10 percent of those under age 65 with incomes over $10,000 per year are unprotected, over 50 percent of those under age 65 with incomes less than $5000 per year have no hospital or surgical insurance at all.

For those who have it, the reimbursement of expenses covered by hospital insurance is limited in many different ways. Overall only 75 percent of consumer expenditures for hospital care are met by private health insurance. For medical care outside the hospital, coverage is considerably more limited. Only 35 percent of the American people under age 65 are covered for doctor's office or home visits, and only 11 percent are covered for dental expenses.

One of the consequences of the distorted pattern of coverage is that hospitals are used for diagnostic tests and for treatment which could have been performed at much less cost on an outpatient basis if the cost had been covered by insurance. Another is that the absence of coverage for out-of-hospital medical care and for preventive care may at times discourage their use. In short, when we talk of "health" insurance, we really mean "sickness" insurance, which in turn usually means "hospitalization" insurance.

Even those covered for a broad range of services frequently find—often at the time of need and not before—that their coverage is far from complete. Overall, only 40 percent of consumer expenditures for medical care are covered by private health insurance. "Deductibles" (the policyholder must pay an initial portion of the cost), "coinsurance" (the policyholder must pay some fraction of the remaining cost) and, one of the most pernicious features of all, overall maximum limitations on the coverage, either in terms of number of services or the total dollar value of the policy, all limit the coverage.

Medicare, the Social Security–based health-insurance program for those over age 65, also includes these types of out-of-pocket liability for the patient, although its coverage (if one includes both Part A, the universal hospitalization coverage, and Part B, the optional ambulatory-care coverage) is better than that of most policies. Since most of the expense is paid through current Social Security payments, the billing for direct premium payments for Medicare is, of course, among the lowest.

Nevertheless, the total out-of-pocket dollar expense for medical care by those over age 65 is now actually *higher* than it was before Medicare was introduced in 1967. In 1966 the average person over 65 paid about $250 out of pocket for care; in 1974 the average was over $400, an increase of 75 percent, considerably more than the 50-percent increase in out-of-pocket expense for those under age 65 during the same period. Much of this increase is due to the general inflation in the economy, but since many of the elderly live on fixed incomes the increase is especially disastrous for them.

While the costs of a catastrophic illness can destroy the lives of those with even the highest incomes, the people generally hit hardest by the personal costs of illness are the so-called medically indigent, people like John van der Sande who are not so poor that they can pass the "means test" for the "charity" of Medicaid (the state-run, partially federally financed program of health insurance for the poor) unless they are willing to use up all that they own in order to reach an arbitrary—and extraordinarily low—definition of eligibility.

Thus the personal high cost of medical care can hurt all groups in the society—the poor who must rely on "charity"; the middle class who are steadily drained by the costs of insurance and direct payments, and may be destroyed by even a moderate illness; and even at times the rich who may find their wealth significantly eroded by a catastrophic illness.

Turning from the sources of the funds to the ways in which

they are spent, the change in distribution from 1929 to 1975 is shown in Figure 7. About 39 percent of total health expenditures are spent on hospital care, 26 percent on professional services (18 percent on physicians' services, 6 percent on dentists' services and 2 percent on "other" services), 9 percent on drugs and 8 percent on nursing homes. Only 2 percent, as we shall explore further in the next section, is spent on governmental public health activities. Specifically, in analyzing the effects of the medical-care system on equity, we must identify the services which cost far more than the others, and identify the specific elements of the medical-care system and the professional group within it which profit far more than others.

Among the high-*cost* (as contrasted with high-profit) elements in the system, the hospital stands almost alone. Hospital costs have risen by far the fastest of all health-care costs. From 1965 to 1975, just the most recent ten years, the cost of a hospital day in the United States trebled. The cost per hospital day in some specialized hospitals in the United States is now over $300, and if the present trends continue, the cost in some will reach $450 per day by 1980. Since the average (mean) length of a hospital stay changed very little, the cost of an average hospital stay also trebled, from about $300 in 1965 to about $900 in 1975. In 1935 approximately 22 percent of national health expenditures was for hospital care; in 1945, 28 percent; in 1955, 32 percent; in 1965, 35 percent; and by 1975, 39 percent.

In the early 1960s the major portion of the increase in costs of hospital care was an increase in payroll costs, which represent approximately two-thirds of hospital expenses. Part of this increase was due—largely as a result of unionization of hospital workers—to a rise in the exceedingly low level of wages of the poorest-paid hospital workers, such as nurses' aides, orderlies and housekeepers. But in the late 1960s and particularly since 1970 the rise in nonpayroll expenses—due in part to the introduction of ever more expensive technology and in part to inflation in the price of goods and services purchased by hospitals—has far outdistanced the rise in payroll expenses.

FIGURE 7

Distribution of National Health Expenditures in the United States, 1929–1975

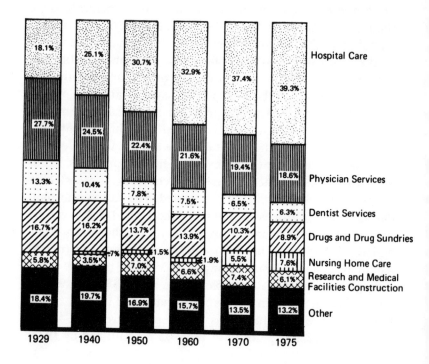

Prepared by the Office of Research and Statistics of the Social Security Administration. The years refer to fiscal years.

Among the high-*profit* elements in the system, drug companies and medical-equipment manufacturers and insurance companies are among the acknowledged leaders, although a few nursing home owners have in recent years provided stiff competition. Annual domestic sales for U.S. drug companies rose from $1.5 billion in 1955 to $6.5 billion in 1974. The average net income-to-sales ratio in the U.S. drug industry in the early 1970s was 9 percent, about twice the industrial median of 4.8 percent, and in some firms the ratio is as high as 18 percent. Even more important to the financial interests of stockholders and the prestige and salaries of managers, the average ratio of net income to invested capital in the industry equaled 17.9 percent, about 50 percent higher than the industrial median of 11.7 percent, and the ratio in individual firms rose as high as 28 percent.

Part of the reason for this is the extremely high prices of many brand-name drugs. One drug company's brand of prednisone, a powerful steroid hormone used in the treatment of arthritis and other illnesses, sold for $102 per 1000 tablets, while a large respectable wholesaler of drugs sold under their generic rather than their brand names sold the same drug under the name prednisone for $4.40 per 1000. These price differentials are largely maintained by patent monopolies and/or by massive advertising campaigns.

Insurance companies make most of their profit in quite a different way. The cash which they hold between the time it is paid in premiums and the time it is paid out in reimbursement for medical expenses constitutes billions of dollars. These funds, together with the billions held for life insurance, fire insurance and other forms of coverage, represent one of the largest pools of capital available in the United States today. A complex, but now thoroughly documented, cross-linkage between the major insurance companies and the major banks permits huge sums to be made—and tremendous power to be wielded—by the use of the incredibly large flow of money that passes through the hands of the insurance companies.

The profits of some nursing home owners are based on what

are in some ways even shabbier—and often illegal—methods. Profits have been made by taking huge sums of money from Medicaid for the care of sick aged people, and then not delivering the services for which they were paid. Mechanisms have included padding of bills, kickbacks, no-show jobs and other forms of frankly criminal behavior. One such owner was alleged to have made a profit of $4.3 million from his nursing homes in a single year. In 1974 another owner was reimbursed at a rate of almost $20,000 for each bed in his nursing home, one of the highest rates in New York State. This rate was paid despite the fact that a New York City Health Department inspection in 1972 found dozens of violations including filth in the kitchen, no recreation for the patients, fire hazards and inadequate nursing staff.

Physicians are by far the highest *income* group in the system. Indeed, physicians as a group are now among the highest-paid people in the United States, and many individual physicians have become notorious for the size of their annual incomes. The 1973 median income for physicians engaged in office-based patient care, after payment of tax-deductible expenses but before payment of income taxes, was $42,140. The income range varied from a high of $51,830 for obstetrician-gynecologists to a "low" of $37,400 for psychiatrists. General surgeons earned the second highest income ($47,290) and internists earned the third highest ($43,000). Many individual physicians net well over $100,000. Incorporated physicians, who, it is estimated, now constitute over one-third of all practicing physicians, earned a median net income in 1973 of $67,500.

In comparison, the median income for all American families in 1973 was $13,373. Among full-time male salaried workers, the median annual earnings in 1973 were: physicians and surgeons, $23,360; engineers and technical personnel, $17,924; and primary and secondary school teachers, $12,019. And there are, of course, huge differences between the income of physicians and other health workers. For example, as discussed later in this chapter, in 1970 the median net income for self-employed doctors in solo practice under age 65 was approximately

$40,000; for pharmacists, $10,000; for technicians and registered nurses, $6,000; and for the lowest-paid service workers, $3,500.

Having analyzed some of the sources of funds for the health- and medical-care system and some of the elements of the distribution of these funds, we can begin to address the question of how great an investment by a society in health care and medical care is "enough." An expenditure of $150 billion or more annually, and of almost one-tenth of our national productivity, sounds, and is, huge. Certainly its distribution, in terms of the pockets from which it came and into which it goes, and, as we shall see, in terms of the services it provides, is indefensible. But the $100 billion spent on health- and medical-care services in 1973 doesn't sound like quite so much when it is compared to the amount that the people of the United States were willing to spend in that year on other items.

Indeed, they spent billions on activities directly inimical to health, including $22 billion for alcoholic beverages, $14 billion for tobacco products and smoker's accessories, and incalculable billions spent on too many automobiles with too much power for the roads they travel (not to speak of too much energy consumption and pollution). Billions were also spent on activities not so clearly inimical to health, including gambling, advertising, cosmetics and pet food—to pick out only a few categories which many people would deem lower in priority than health care and medical care.

The amount spent on health also pales when compared with the billions of late-1970s dollars already allocated for new military helicopters and development work on the B-1 bomber, or the $25 billion asked by the Pentagon for the actual production of 244 B-1 bombers. It shrinks even further in comparison with the 675 billion less-deflated dollars of the 1960s spent by the United States on the Indochina War and compared to the estimated $1.4 trillion spent by the United States on military forces since the end of World War II.

Of course a society's expenditures, if spent inside the country, are also its income, the wages of its workers. Health- and medical-care expenditures now are—and if more equitably distributed could be even more—an important way for people to earn a living in the United States. The question, in short, for a wealthy country like the United States, is not so much "How much are we spending?" but rather "Out of whose pockets does it come?" "Into whose pockets does it go?" "What do we get for it?" and "What are we willing to give up for it?" To give up education or police and fire protection for medical care is unthinkable; to give up or lessen our use of tobacco and alcohol, trips to the moon, environmentally dangerous automobiles, bombers, and wars against small Asian countries may be not only thinkable but even socially useful.

4. Despite—and perhaps in part because of—the vast resources devoted to it, the U.S. medical-care system pays little attention to preventive medicine or rehabilitation, and what it does provide is inequitably distributed.

At the beginning of this century, six of the ten leading causes of death in the United States, including the top three causes, were infectious diseases or closely related to infectious diseases. At the present time only two of the ten leading causes of death are related to infections: "influenza and pneumonia," which ranks sixth, and "diseases of infancy" (only some of which are infectious), which ranks seventh. And the death rates from these causes are far lower than they were in 1900. It is widely agreed that the fall in incidence of many serious infectious diseases is largely due to changes in environmental conditions and the application of public health measures. But the medical-care system has also played a role—in the immunization of individual patients and in the treatment of patients ill with infectious diseases.

Today the list of causes of death is headed by heart disease, cancer and cerebrovascular disease (stroke)—all chronic diseases or the complications of chronic disease. The death rates for the first two have each increased by about 250 percent since 1900. Other chronic diseases, such as diabetes and cirrhosis of the liver, have also emerged as leading causes of death. Of every 100 males born in the United States this year, over 85 are destined to die eventually of a chronic disease; in 1900 the rate was closer to 50 in 100 births.

Again, death rates are only a part of the story, particularly for chronic illnesses since they may afflict large numbers of the living for long periods of time. Heart and circulatory disorders may today be present in as many as 30 million Americans, disabling mental and emotional disorders in 20 million, and arthritis and rheumatic diseases in 16 million. Infectious diseases usually have a fairly abrupt onset and, with some exceptions, a finite duration. Recognition by the patient of their presence and of their severity, through fever, pain, cough or other symptoms, is usually rapid, consultation with the medical-care system is usually prompt, and (except for viral illnesses, which are for the most part self-limited) treatment is usually quite specific and effective. Chronic diseases, on the other hand, typically have a gradual onset and an indefinite duration. Patients with cancer or heart disease, emphysema or glaucoma, diabetes or cirrhosis, may be developing progressive illness and complications for months or even years before they realize that they are afflicted.

Patients with these two very different types of illness have very different needs and make different demands on a health-care system. For many infectious diseases, with important exceptions like tuberculosis or venereal disease, it may be acceptable in the care of the patient to wait until the patient comes to the doctor with symptoms, although prevention or early detection, and hence prevention of spread to others, is of course preferable where possible. For many chronic diseases, however, like glaucoma, hypertension and some forms of cancer, discovering the presence of the illness early, before symptoms begin, may be an important factor in the later course of the illness. For infectious disease, treatment is usually directed at a causative organism; for chronic illness, treatment is often directed at the symptoms rather than at the cause. In infectious diseases, one may usually hope for cure; in chronic illness, the goal is more often care rather than cure.

Here it is important to note that the chronically ill patient must usually be far more involved as a manager in the care of his own illness than is necessary or perhaps even possible for the patient who has a short-lived infectious disease; the latter individual is often acutely, if temporarily, incapacitated and dependent. But the patient with a chronic disease is at many important stages of the illness more or less able to go about his or her normal business, and this may interfere with current patterns of medical care which are based on the convenience of the doctor or the institution. The care of chronic illness is by definition protracted, and often extremely costly. A system geared to one-to-one, episodic, fee-for-individual-service relationships is unwieldy, inefficient and often self-defeating when the patient requires integrated, comprehensive care by many different types of doctors and by many different types of health workers, including nurses, therapists and social workers, and often by many different institutions over a period of months or years.

The U.S. medical-care system has in the main ignored preventive medicine in general and these changing needs for prevention and care in particular. Each year the portion of national "health" expenditures spent on medical care for those who are already ill—particularly technological care in the hospital—grows larger and the portion spent on health protection grows smaller. As we have seen, public health activities by all levels of government accounted for only about 2 percent of the nation's health expenditures. Even if one includes services for health protection provided through nongovernmental funds, the total is almost certainly less than 5 percent. In short, almost ten times as much is spent on care in the hospital alone and, overall, some twenty times as much is spent trying to cure or care for the ill as on trying to prevent illness and promote health.

In order to analyze in greater depth the provision of health care, it is useful to classify preventive measures by the three levels in the natural history of disease at which they can be applied. The first level, technically called "primary prevention," is that of promoting health and preventing the basic disease process from taking hold in the person at all. Examples include promotion of measures likely to lead to better health, such as cessation of smoking and elimination of environmental pollution; control of industrial hazards to prevent occupational accidents and illness; provision of uncontaminated foods and water so as to prevent acute and chronic infections; immunization against specific types of infectious disease; and fluoridation of water supplies to prevent dental cavities.

The next level of prevention, called "secondary prevention," attempts to halt or to reverse a disease process once it has begun, in order to prevent its consequences and complications. Examples include the lowering of high blood pressure to prevent strokes, kidney failure and heart failure; or the detection of a breast cancer while it is still localized so it can be treated before it has spread to other parts of the body.

The third level of prevention, called "tertiary prevention," consists of preventing, and if possible reversing, the deterioration of the quality of life due to a chronic illness or disability. This includes formal rehabilitation and retraining where possible and teaching the patient how to cope successfully with the disability.

At all of these levels, preventive care in the United States is seriously deficient. In primary prevention, for example, levels of immunization against infectious disease lag far behind those of other affluent countries, and the level of protection is lowest among the poor. In a recent outbreak of diphtheria in San Antonio those most affected were the city's chicano and black population, who had rates over ten times that of the white population. Safe and effective immunization exists for this disease, usually given to infants in combination with immunization against whooping cough (pertussis) and tetanus. The poor of San Antonio were both at the greatest risk of exposure to diphtheria and had the lowest levels of protection against it.

Even diseases that have been "conquered" provide examples of the grossest forms of inequity during the process of conquest. While poliomyelitis (infantile paralysis) was still widespread in the United States, the virus could be encountered in swimming holes and elsewhere in the childhood environment of the poor. Paralytic polio, as contrasted with a milder nonparalytic form, often spared those children who because of their poverty had had early exposure to the virus and were naturally immunized by having had a mild form of the illness early in life. Paralytic polio was therefore largely concentrated among the upper classes, who lacked this early environmental exposure to the virus. Franklin Delano Roosevelt, of course, was one of its best-known adult victims.

As early natural exposure of children to the virus was reduced through environmental improvement, and as the polio vaccine was introduced inequitably—largely through private doctors—into the United States, the pattern of paralytic polio changed dramatically. The children of the affluent were protected by immunization, obtained through their private pediatricians; the children of the poor were often unprotected, without "benefit" of either early natural exposure or immunization. As a result the paralytic polio epidemics of the late 1950s largely struck the poor. This was a transient phenomenon, since extremely few new cases of paralytic polio occur in the United States at the present time, but the low current levels of immunization mean that the potential for future disaster continues.

Another area of primary prevention that is widely felt to be deficient in the United States is that of prevention of accidents and of occupation-related illnesses.

It has been estimated that approximately 14,000 lives—more than 25 percent of the annual motor vehicle fatalities—could be saved if everyone simply wore seat belts or if automatic restraints such as air bags were universally introduced. Yet measures such as these have been consistently resisted in the United States.

In addition over 15,000 American workers are killed each

year in work accidents, over 100,000 die of work-related diseases, and over two million are either permanently or temporarily disabled as a result of work accidents and occupational disease. State laws governing occupational safety standards are uneven and poorly enforced. Federal laws are weak and unenforced; there are so few federal inspectors of occupational health and safety that a workplace in the United States can only be inspected on the average *once every 20 years,* and even when violations of safety and health standards are found, often only a slap on the wrist—such as a small fine—is administered.

Household accidents kill 30,000 people a year. Chemical pollutants pour into the air and water. It has been estimated that some 80 percent of the cancer in the United States is caused by environmental factors.

Yet few American physicians—and few medical-care workers of any sort—see it as part of their responsibilities to work for occupational or motor vehicle or household safety, or even to raise their voices about the perils of environmental pollution.

Another aspect of primary prevention is related to habits and life-style. A long-term study in California investigated the relationship between mortality and seven characteristics: exercising regularly; maintaining moderate weight in relation to height; eating breakfast; not snacking between meals; avoiding smoking; limiting liquor consumption; and sleeping at least seven hours a night. The "life expectancy" for men at age 45 who maintained six or seven of these habits was on the average *11 years* longer than the "life expectancy" for men who maintained three or less of them.

Remarkably little effort is expended in educating people about such findings and persuading them to act for the protection of their own health. Despite a decrease in the last decade in the proportion of adult men who smoke, almost 40 percent still do; and there has been almost no change in the proportion of adult females who smoke—about 30 percent. Even more disturbing, there has been no decline in cigarette smoking among teen-agers; in fact, there has been an *increase* in smoking among female teen-agers. Furthermore, about 40 percent of adult males and 16 percent of adult females are moderate-to-heavy drinkers, and an estimated nine million Americans are alcoholics or "problem drinkers." Drinking among teen-agers is now extremely widespread; 36 percent of high-school students report getting drunk at least four times a year.

Yet another area of preventive medicine, usually combining both primary and secondary prevention, is prenatal care. A study sponsored by the Institute of Medicine of the National Academy of Sciences recently analyzed the medical risks and social conditions during pregnancy, the medical care, and the survival history of all of the babies born in New York City in 1968. The study demonstrated that good prenatal care is indeed associated with a greater chance of infant survival. It also showed that pregnant women with the greatest medical and social problems had the least adequate care. Of the 22,000 black and Puerto Rican mothers at "social risk," *less than 2 percent* had what the consultants to the Institute of Medicine defined as adequate care. That figure is so shocking it deserves repetition: Fewer than 1 in 50 of the high-risk black and Puerto Rican pregnant women in New York City had adequate care—and that was before the New York City fiscal crisis forced massive cutbacks in medical care for the poor of the city.

With regard to secondary prevention, there is somewhat more effort, but still minuscule in relation to the total resources devoted to health and medical care. Some valid community screening programs, such as those for hypertension, do exist, but it is nonetheless estimated that about half of the approximately 23 million people with hypertension in the United States are unaware of their ticking time bomb. Extensive regular physical "checkups" are urged by some physicians, although the value of all but a few of the tests has been seriously called into question. The checkup has been criticized as designed more to contribute to physicians' incomes than to find early signs of illness but some elements are clearly useful.

In the United Kingdom, where the individual has easy access to a primary-care physician at no cost at the time of care, and where it is therefore often easier to recognize dangerous symptoms when they first occur, the "checkup" is rarely used and generally condemned. In the United States, where access to a primary-care physician is often more difficult, and costly, where the individual often does not have an ongoing relationship with a physician, and where dramatic technological diagnostic methods are often preferred over continuing observation of the patient, the patient is made to feel guilty if he does not have an annual checkup, which generally relies heavily on mechanical means of assessing health.

For those screening examinations which are indeed thought to be of importance in secondary prevention, there are huge gaps in performance. Relatively simple procedures, such as teaching women how to examine their own breasts for the presence of new or growing lumps, and educating people on what symptoms may suggest dangerous but potentially reversible illness, are neglected by all but a few physicians and health agencies.

Regular physical examination of children is felt to be especially important because growth problems and other defects can be found while something can still be done about them. Yet the National Health Interview Survey in 1973 found that over one-third of children under the age of 17 had had no physical examination within the previous two years. In this area as well, the poor are less likely than the affluent to receive the benefits of preventive medicine. The rate of physical examination is 30 percent higher among children in families with incomes of $15,000 or more per year than among children in families earning $5000 per year or less.

What makes this differential shocking is that poor children were specifically made eligible for such examinations, and for any follow-up treatment that proved to be required, under the Medicaid program. Yet an October 1976 House of Representatives subcommittee report, entitled "Shortchanging Children," reveals that of 12.9 million young people under the age of 21 who were eligible for medical examinations and treatment under Medicaid in 1975, 10.9 million (85 percent) were neither examined nor treated. The subcommittee estimated, for example, that about one million of the unscreened children would have needed treatment or care for a perceptual deficiency, including 650,000 with eye defects.

Helping people to rehabilitate themselves, or to cope successfully with their chronic illnesses so as to prevent unnecessary disability, is an equally neglected area of prevention. Billions of dollars are spent on nursing homes, but only a small portion of that is spent on rehabilitation. What is done, rather, has been aptly termed "warehousing" the chronically ill or the elderly. At the other extreme is the application of technological models which may be ill-suited, ineffective and dangerous for the patient whose most pressing need is for methods of coping with his or her own illness, and for family and community support in those activities of life which have become difficult or impossible due to the chronic illness. In fact, the medical-care system—presumably without conscious intent—often converts chronic illness, which it cannot handle, into an acute illness, such as an adverse drug reaction, an infection or an operative complication, which it does know how to deal with.

Among the successful methods for helping people to understand and cope with chronic illness have been self-help groups, such as mastectomy clubs or colostomy clubs, and other community support systems. Yet these have not only received little attention or support from the medical-care system but are often viewed with disdain as being outside the professional aegis.

5. But the massive investment in therapeutic medicine also fails to meet our needs: The U.S. medical-care system is fragmented; has large amounts of public financing, yet little public accountability; is devoted largely to technology and relatively little to care; and is grossly maldistributed geographically and socially.

Although in one sense the U.S. medical-care system is highly structured—for the benefit of those who control it and of some of those who work in it—in another sense it is so fragmented, the responsibilities so diffuse, the levels of control so manifold, the communication and coordination between its parts so haphazard, that—except for the euphemisms "pluralistic" and "pragmatic"—the system almost defies brief description.

One type of analysis, analogous in some ways to the classifications of levels of prevention, is the definition of various levels of care as "primary," "secondary" and "tertiary" according to the severity of the illness and the nature of the medical response that is required.

At the first level, the patient with relatively minor symptoms or who is worried about his health may seek reassurance or care in a number of different ways. Self-care, often with medications available without prescription ("over the counter"), is the most frequent response to common symptoms or anxiety which an individual feels on a given day. Such an individual may turn to members of his family for advice and care, or to nonprofessional people within his community. Teachers or fellow workers are often consulted on various types of health problems. In some cultures spiritualists, herbalists or other well-defined individuals within the culture are consulted at times of minor illness, or even illness of greater severity.

The first contact with the professional medical system is often with a professional other than a physician. Pharmacists, for example, play an important role in first-contact professional care. If a physician is to be consulted as the point of first-contact professional care, the choice of the type of physician to be contacted is quite different from country to country. In most countries the physician of first contact will be a "primary-care physician," which, as we define the term, signifies a physician based in the community rather than in a hospital; a physician people first turn to, who does not regularly see referrals from other physicians; who provides continuing care rather than episodic care; and who serves the function of integrating the work of referral specialists and other community resources in relation to the patient's care.

In this sequence, "secondary care" is that which is provided by specialists, either on an ambulatory basis or in the hospital, and "tertiary care" is that which is provided in specialized hospitals by highly specialized or subspecialized personnel. In the United States, however, first-contact primary care is often provided by specialists, by emergency rooms and by hospital outpatient departments—resources which in other societies are largely reserved for secondary or even tertiary care.

Beyond these three levels of medical care is that of long-term care for the chronically ill or disabled. In the United States, long-term care is often provided in chronic hospitals or in nursing homes for those whose illnesses are so severe that function outside of an institution is impossible or, in an increasing number of instances, for those who have no alternative place with either family or friends in which they can be given the care they need while continuing to function within the society.

Another framework for analysis is based on the nature of the controlling institution. These institutions are usually divided into three basic groups, one conventionally defined as "public" (meaning governmental) and two defined as "private," although the distinctions increasingly have less and less meaning.

Let us begin with the elements of the system in the "public" sector. All levels of government play a role in health care and in medical care, with a complex mix of direct operating responsibility for some elements, funding for others, and regulation for yet others. The federal government directly *operates* medical-care delivery programs for military personnel and their families, for veterans and for native Americans on reservations. It *finances* medical care for the aged and for a limited group of other disabled people through Medicare and indirectly pays a major part of the cost of medical care for the poor through Medicaid; it is the major funding agency for the construction of medical facilities and for medical research; and it provides a large part of the funding for medical education directly to medical schools and indirectly through scholarships and loan funds for medical students. Finally, the federal government has important *regulatory* authority over health and medical affairs involving "interstate commerce," such as food and drugs, occupational health and safety, and environmental pollution. Overall, federal money accounts for nearly 30 percent of all U.S.

health expenditures. These include about 25 percent of all funds spent on personal health and medical-care services, 65 percent of the investment in biomedical research and development, and over 45 percent of the revenues of the nation's medical schools.

State governments provide medical care directly for many of the mentally ill and, until recently, those with tuberculosis; they administer and contribute to the financing of health care for the poor through Medicaid; they conduct statewide public health programs; they operate medical schools, usually through a state university, and contribute to the financing of others; and they license hospitals and a wide range of health workers.

Local governments, at the county and municipal levels, often provide inpatient and ambulatory-care services directly for the poor. They also carry out a wide variety of public health functions, including the collecting of vital statistics and statistics on reportable illnesses; controlling communicable diseases, including tuberculosis and venereal diseases; monitoring environmental sanitation, including water quality and supervision of foods and eating places; providing maternal and child health services, including school health services; and conducting programs of health education.

In short, almost all "public health services" in the United States and many personal medical-care services are directly provided by government agencies, and many other personal medical-care services are financed by government.

The two parts of the "private" sector are defined as "profit-making" (sometimes called, for historical reasons, "proprietary" or, for public-relations reasons, "investor-owned") and "nonprofit-making" (sometimes termed "voluntary" or "eleemosynary").

Examples of parts of the system almost entirely in the profit-making sector are nursing homes; pharmaceutical research, manufacture, distribution and sale; and commercial health-insurance companies. For the United States as a whole, most ambulatory medical and dental care is in the profit-making part of the private sector, although the situation is different in the centers of some of our largest cities where many of these services are provided by government or by voluntary hospitals.

Only a small fraction of U.S. hospital beds lie in profit-making hospitals, many of which are owned by groups of physicians.

The "nonprofit" sector includes the voluntary hospitals, which contain over 60 percent of the country's acute-general-care beds; many of the nation's medical schools, including some of its most prestigious ones; and insurance organizations in each state affiliated with each other under the name of Blue Cross and Blue Shield, providing insurance respectively for hospitalization costs and for doctors' fees.

In sum, a large part of the U.S. medical-care system—as contrasted with its health-care system—is controlled by the private sector, even though, as we have seen, large amounts of it are financed publicly. Furthermore, the fact that medical care is largely controlled by the private sector and that health care is largely controlled by the public sector is surely one of the major reasons for the overwhelmingly greater investment in treatment rather than in prevention. This is especially true for ambulatory care. Of the 1.1 billion patient visits made annually in the United States (an average of five visits per person per year), two-thirds are made to private medical practitioners and private group practices, almost all on a fee-for-service basis. Another 18 percent of the visits nationwide—though a far higher percent in the inner cities—are made to hospital outpatient departments and emergency rooms, many of them also in the "private" (albeit "nonprofit") sector.

The situation shifts markedly when one looks at inpatient hospital care. Mainly because of the large number of long-stay beds in mental hospitals owned by state and local governments, and to a lesser extent the number of beds in the federal government's Veterans Administration, Armed Services, and Public Health Service hospitals, approximately half the U.S. hospital beds are in government-owned and -operated hospitals. Only 5 percent of the beds are in proprietary hospitals, owned and operated for profit. The remaining 45 percent are in voluntary hospitals, operated on a nonprofit basis by churches, other organized groups, or by self-elected and self-perpetuated boards of trustees.

It is of interest that since 1946 the ratio of hospital beds of all kinds to population has decreased, from one bed for every 100 people to one for every 130 people. The decrease has occurred largely in federal hospitals and in psychiatric, tuberculosis and other long-term hospitals. At the same time, however, there has been an increase in the bed/population ratio for short-term general hospitals. There are now approximately 4.5 short-term general medical and surgical beds per 1000 population (one for every 225 people); of these, in contrast to the situation for long-stay beds, only about one-third are operated by government. There has also been a trend over this period to larger hospitals, with a reduction in the number of hospitals having less than 100 beds. Despite the fact that hospitals have increased in size in the name of efficiency and despite the net movement of people from rural areas to metropolitan areas where hospitals are larger, the level of bed occupancy has changed almost not at all from 1946 (75 percent) to 1975 (76 percent).

The training and practice of the health workers in the system are also fragmented and there is little accountability to the public. Patterns for education of physicians are largely set by nongovernmental bodies, such as the Association of American Medical Colleges, and by the medical schools themselves. Although there is an increasing attempt at coordination of criteria for licensure and the use of a standardized national examination, licensure standards are set on a state-by-state basis, almost in every case by physician-dominated boards with little public accountability. Except for the internal standards set by hospitals and other medical institutions, which vary widely and are often unenforced, any physician, whatever his or her training, can legally do anything in medical practice: perform neurosurgery, counsel people with marital problems or read X rays. For physicians who practice largely outside institutions, fear of malpractice suits is almost the only deterrent—other than conscience—to undertaking procedures in which they have had only minimal training or experience.

Of the approximately 375,000 active physicians in the United States (one for every 550 people), almost 8 percent are employed by the federal government and approximately 20 percent are in salaried hospital practice; some of the former and most of the latter are in training programs, usually as interns and residents. Approximately another 10 percent are employed in teaching, administration, research and other activities not directly related to patient care. The remaining 60 percent of active doctors are employed in "office-based" patient care, most of them practicing on a fee-for-service basis.

Physicians are largely free to choose their own form of post-graduate training and their own form of practice. As a result over the past quarter-century there has been a major shift away from primary care—first-contact, continuing integrated care for the patient—and a major shift toward specialist practice, as shown in Figure 8. Even if one includes doctors who say they "limit their practice" to internal medicine and pediatrics, the supply of primary-care doctors in the United States has fallen sharply from 1930, when there was approximately one for every 1000 people, to 1970, when there was one for every 2000.

There has been somewhat of a reversal in the 1970s, due in part to the efforts of the federal and state governments, but the number of specialist physicians still far exceeds the number of primary-care physicians. In fact, the United States probably exceeds all other countries in the world in the extent to which medical care is given by physicians who consider themselves specialists rather than generalists or even, as is the increasing trend in the United States, as "specialists" in "family practice."

The result, of course, of this specialization and of the benefit coverage of most health-insurance policies, which cover hospital care but rarely ambulatory care and even more rarely continuing and preventive care, is a medical-care system devoted largely to technological diagnosis and treatment for serious acute illness and relatively little to care for less serious acute illness and to care for chronic illness and disability.

Similar kinds of analyses can be applied to nurses and other health workers. Among the major differences is that most nurses, for example, are salaried rather than fee-for-service entrepreneurs, that a far higher percentage of them are women, and that their incomes are far lower than those of doctors. But there are also vast similarities: a fragmentation of training pat-

FIGURE 8

Distribution of Physicians by Specialization Status
in the United States, 1949–1972

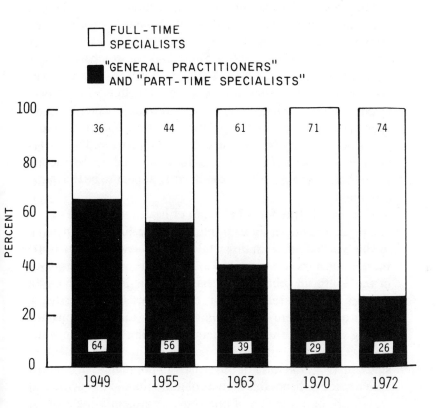

Modified by the authors from a figure prepared by the University of Michigan
School of Public Health from data published by the U.S. Public Health Service
(before 1970) and the National Center for Health Statistics (1970 and 1972).
The data include only M.D.s in private practice.

terns with little public control, an increasing emphasis in training (the "university-trained" nurse) and in practice (the "nurse-clinician") on technology rather than care, and gross geographic and social maldistribution.

The gross maldistribution of health workers in the United States can be seen by a regional, a state-by-state, or a community-by-community analysis. In 1973 there was, for example, one doctor for every 1343 people in South Dakota, compared to one for every 432 people in New York, as shown in Figure 9. The differences among states are not simply a result of differences in population density; Vermont and Iowa, for example, have approximately the same population density, but there is one physician for every 565 people in Vermont compared to one for every 999 in Iowa. The wealth of the state, and its desirability to physicians as a place to live and work, appear to be the major attractions.

The same is true for other types of health workers. There is one registered nurse, for example, for every 400 to 500 persons in the South Central states while in the New England states there is one nurse for every 150 to 200 people; an average person in the South, in other words, has available less than half the number of nurses than does his counterpart in the Northeast.

Not only is there gross maldistribution among regions and among states, but there is similar maldistribution within states and within cities. In a study performed in the Appalachian states in 1967, the ratio of physicians to population in counties with a median disposable income of more than $5000 per family was, with the exception of one state, consistently higher than the ratio in counties with an income of $5000 or less per family (Figure 10). In Maryland, Tennessee and Alabama, for example, there were almost three times as many doctors per capita in the rich counties as in the poor counties, and in Virginia, West Virginia and North Carolina, there were about twice as many per capita for the wealthy counties as for the poor.

Individual small, relatively isolated communities often have severe difficulty in recruiting or in keeping a physician. The National Health Service Corps estimated in 1976 that there

FIGURE 9

Ratio of Physicians to Population by State, 1970

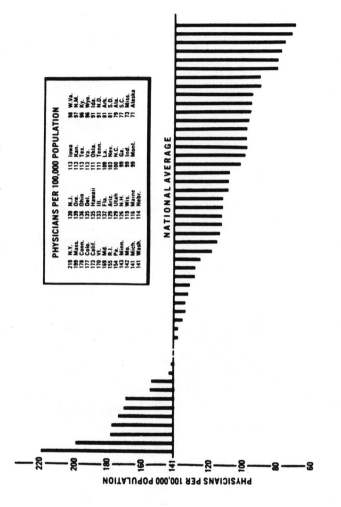

PHYSICIANS PER 100,000 POPULATION

219 N.Y.	139 N.J.	113 Iowa
199 Mass.	139 Ore.	113 Kan.
178 Conn.	136 Ohio	113 Tex.
177 Colo.	135 Del.	113 Va.
173 Calif.	135 Hawaii	111 Okla.
170 Vt.	133 Ill.	111 Tenn.
169 Md.	132 Fla.	109 La.
155 R.I.	129 Ariz.	103 Nev.
154 Pa.	129 Utah	100 N.C.
143 Minn.	126 N.H.	99 Ga.
142 Mo.	119 Wis.	99 Ind.
141 Mich.	116 Maine	99 Mont.
141 Wash.	114 Nebr.	

98 W.Va.	
97 N.M.	
96 Ky.	
96 Wyo.	
91 Ida.	
91 N.D.	
81 Ark.	
81 S.D.	
79 Ala.	
77 S.C.	
73 Miss.	
71 Alaska	

NATIONAL AVERAGE

PHYSICIANS PER 100,000 POPULATION

220 — 200 — 180 — 160 — 141 — 120 — 100 — 80 — 60

Published by the U.S. Department of Health, Education and Welfare, 1971.

FIGURE 10

Ratio of Physicians to Population in the Appalachian States, by Wealth of County, 1967

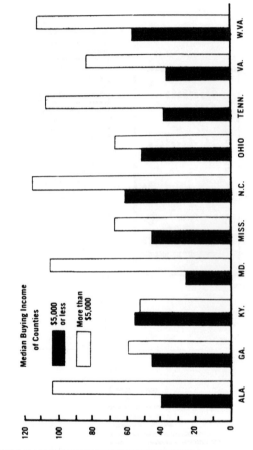

Published by the U.S. Department of Health, Education and Welfare, 1971.

were 748 U.S. communities that lacked a physician. These doc-
torless communities were located in 46 states; every one of the
United States, with the exception of Hawaii, Massachusetts,
New Jersey and Rhode Island, had at least one town needing
a doctor.

Inside the large cities the maldistribution of physicians is
equally severe, but it is harder to demonstrate statistically because many of the teaching hospitals, with their large numbers
of doctors, are located in the midst of what have become the
poorest urban areas. However, because they limit their practice
to specialties or subspecialties or because they are in training for
these specialties, most of these hospital-based doctors are unavailable to meet the general medical-care needs of the poor who
surround them. A study performed in Boston, for example,
showed that the number of general-care physicians per capita
was twice as high in affluent areas studied as in poor ones.

Even when general-care doctors are available—often grudg-
ingly—in outpatient departments and in the emergency rooms
of the hospitals (and, because of the inaccessibility of general
medical care elsewhere, the emergency room is becoming the
place in which much primary medical care is currently being
given), there are great barriers to access by the poor. Members
of the New York City Department of Health in the mid-1960s
described some of the remaining barriers, even when those
imposed by cost of care are removed, which keep poor people
from equitable access to medical care. These include inadequate
transportation, complex and imposing institutions, difficulty in
taking time off from work or in finding someone to take care
of the children, and the fragmentation and repeated visits common in such care.

Medicaid, which was intended to ameliorate some of the
inequity of access, has indeed brought physicians into the urban
ghetto, but the nature of the financial incentives which brought
them in have led to other forms of abuse. One is the promotion
of brief and unnecessarily frequent visits, with the "ping-pong-
ing" of patients from one physician to other, often in a shared
facility known as a "Medicaid mill." This is done so that each

physician may charge a separate fee for the partial service rendered. For the same reason—receipt of extra fees—the number of lab tests and number of prescriptions seem far in excess of the number needed. There are exceptions, of course, both among some principled and therefore in fact self-sacrificing individual doctors operating in fee-for-service practice and in those few instances where Medicaid has been used to support forms of practice different from fee-for-service care.

Paradoxically, programs like Medicaid themselves produce limited access to care, due to their reimbursement levels and their bureaucratic structure. Patients in New York State are required to reregister for Medicaid monthly, no matter how sick or how poor they are. Delays of up to six months or longer in payments to providers of care are common, and limitations on reimbursement often have little or no relationship to actual costs, causing many physicians, pharmacists and other providers to refuse to accept Medicaid patients.

Overall, the poor in the United States actually average slightly more physician visits per year than do the more affluent. In 1973, for example, people aged 17–44 with family income under $6000 per year averaged 5.7 physician visits per year, while those with incomes of $6000 or more in this age group averaged 5.0 visits. This indeed represents a substantial shift toward the poor in number of visits from 1964, when for the same age group there were 4.1 visits per year among the poor (defined then as having family income less than $3000) and 4.7 visits among the "nonpoor."

Compared to their health-care needs, however, visits to physicians by the poor would have to be far higher for there to be equitable distribution of physician resources. (See Figures 11 and 12.) We have already discussed the findings in the National Health Interview Survey among people aged 17–44 which show that the poor have much more disease and disability than do the affluent. Yet despite the fact that the medical-care needs of the poor in this age group would seem to be far greater than the needs of the affluent, their average annual rate of visits to physicians is less than 20 percent higher.

FIGURE 11

Restricted Activity and Bed Disability Days
per Person per Year, by Family Income, 1971

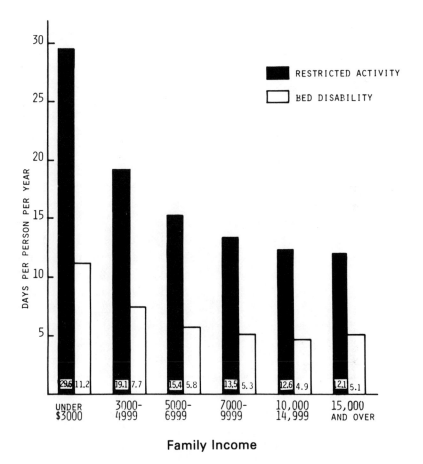

Figure prepared by the University of Michigan School of Public Health from data published by the National Center for Health Statistics. The data are limited to the civilian, noninstitutionalized population of the United States.

FIGURE 12

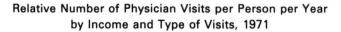

Relative Number of Physician Visits per Person per Year
by Income and Type of Visits, 1971

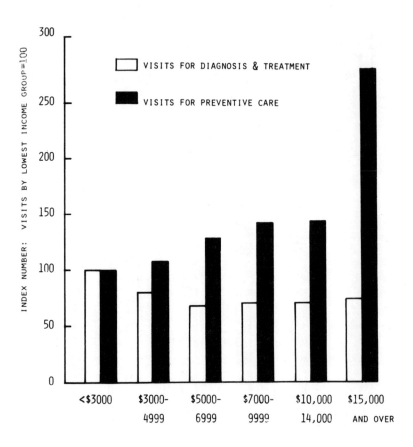

Family Income

Figure prepared by the University of Michigan School of Public Health from
data published by the National Center for Health Statistics.

If one looks at the 45–64 age group, the difference between the obvious needs of the poor and the needs of the affluent for medical care is even greater; yet in this age group the actual differential between rich and poor in average rate of physician visits is approximately the same as for the younger group. For hospitalization, however, the differential use between the rich and the poor does seem to reflect somewhat equitably their grossly different medical-care needs.

Only at ages greater than 65, where the number of medical problems for *both* the rich and the poor are far greater and where Medicare—administered, unlike Medicaid, through federal standards rather than state standards—has indeed made access more equitable, do the needs for care and the use of care seem to even out somewhat. For the elderly the inequity in use of medical care rests more in comparison with the young in the population. For example, those over age 65 of all incomes have almost twice as much arthritis, diabetes and hypertension as those in the 45–64 age group and almost three times as much hearing and vision impairment; they have almost three times as many bed disability days; and there are four times as many with limitation of mobility. Yet the average number of physician visits per year for the elderly is only 20 percent higher (6.5 visits per year compared to 5.5 visits per year) than for those aged 44–64.

Furthermore, taking all age groups together, as in Figures 11 and 12, not only do the rates of visits for diagnosis and treatment appear not to reflect the relative medical-care needs of the poor, but the rates of visits for preventive care, as discussed in Section 4, are far higher for the affluent than for the poor.

For specific groups of people defined in other ways, the lack of equity in use of care is even more striking. Looking again at those aged 17–44, but now differentiating between those the National Health Interview Survey classified as "white" and those it classified "all other" (*i.e.,* "nonwhite"), there is twice as much diabetes and hypertension, at least 30 percent more restricted-activity days, bed disability days and work-loss days, and some 60 percent more limitation in mobility among the "nonwhite" population than among the "white." Yet "nonwhites" in this age group actually have *fewer* physician visits per year than do the "whites."

These discrepancies are startling enough, but become even more striking if one examines where the visits take place. For example, again for the 17–44 age group, for the "whites" 5.6 percent of the physician visits were to hospital outpatient clinics and 4.0 percent were to emergency rooms; for the "nonwhites," almost three times the percentage (13.4 percent) were to OPDs and almost twice the percentage (7.3 percent) were to hospital emergency rooms.

Anyone familiar with the differences (in general; there are exceptions) in comfort, in waiting time and in the humanity of the experience between being seen in a physician's or group's office and being seen in a hospital OPD or ER will understand what these dry statistics represent in the nature of the contact with medical care. But the statistics reflect not only disparities in comfort and convenience, they also represent vast differences in continuity and consistency of care and in the attention paid to preventive medicine, with the "nonwhites"—and the poor of all colors—with rare exceptions getting by far the less continuity and the less preventive medicine.

Interestingly, the distribution of hospital beds in the United States is much more equitable than that of physicians. In 1948 some states had as few as two general medical and surgical hospital beds per 1000 population. Since that year, however, the Hill-Burton program, a federal hospital-construction program, has spent more than $12 billion, in addition to even greater amounts of local funds, for hospital construction and modernization. As a result of these vast expenditures the distribution of hospital beds throughout the country has become much more balanced. States such as Mississippi, Alabama, Georgia and Tennessee, which had the lowest bed/population ratios in 1948, are now at the national average or above it. Some of the states with particularly high bed/population ratios in 1948 have experienced a decrease, and within states there is also evidence of a more equitable distribution of hospital facilities between rich and poor areas. In some ways hospital-bed distribution is used to "make up for" shortages of physicians; states, like South Dakota, which have low physician-to-population ratios, have relatively high hospital bed/population ratios. While part of the object of the Hill-Burton program was to "lure" physicians into rural areas by building hospitals there, the strategy has largely been a failure.

There is indeed gross maldistribution and social misuse of hospital resources, but it takes a different form than that of physicians and other health workers. The maldistribution and misuse occur in the competition among hospitals, particularly in urban areas, for prestige-enhancing equipment and for patients to keep the beds full.

Examples of needless and dangerous duplication of expensive equipment are ubiquitous. It was estimated in 1971, for example, that the number of teletherapy units (containing X-ray equipment used for treating certain kinds of cancer) concentrated on Chicago's near-South Side could, if properly distributed, take care of the needs of the entire state of Illinois. There were teletherapy units in Chicago that had never even been used since their installation because no one knew how to operate the equipment. Furthermore, the Chicago Regional Hospital Study estimated that a more rational distribution of teletherapy and coronary-care units might cut the operating costs of Chicago hospitals by as much as 10 percent.

The most commonly cited examples of expensive and hazardous duplication of services lie in the field of open-heart surgery, in which complex and costly heart-lung machines are used to maintain the patient's blood flow while surgeons repair or replace valves or other parts of the heart. The duplication of such units is so extensive that, despite intense competition for patients, many hospitals manage to attract only a few candidates for such surgery and thus perform extremely few such operations. The Inter-Society Commission for Heart Disease Resources reported that in 1969, 360 U.S. hospitals were equipped to do open-heart surgery. Of these, 220 average 50 operations or less a year—less than one per week. The commission, composed of experts in heart disease, advises that an open-heart surgery unit can maintain its skills and function efficiently only if it does a minimum of 200 operations a year, a minimum of 4 on the average per week. Of the 360 U.S. hospitals with units, only 15 actually performed 200 or more in 1969.

Not only is the proliferation of open-heart units costly, but it is also murderous. The evidence for unnecessary deaths recently reported at a hospital outside Boston has already been described earlier in this chapter.

The most recent rush to duplicate facilities has been for computed tomographic (CT) scanners which can diagnose conditions that previously could only be found by exploratory surgery or other invasive techniques. The machines cost an average of $500,000 to purchase and install and $100,000 annually to run. In mid-1976 there were over 300 CT scanners in operation in the United States and over 500 more approved for installation. The hospital portion of the private sector is now under some control by federally mandated Health Systems Agencies and other hospital planning bodies, so the hospital competition is somewhat constrained. Private offices and group practices are not so constrained and there is some evidence that an extraordinarily expensive piece of technology will move into areas of use in which there is even less quality and utilization control than in hospitals; almost 20 percent of CT installations are already in private offices.

In short, the fragmentation and the lack of accountability of the U.S. medical-care system have led to severe inequities, inefficiency and danger. In all areas of medical care, with the possible exception of hospitalization, the poor and nonwhite, who by almost every measure have far greater needs for care than do the more affluent, have less than equitable access to medical care. And the duplications and overlapping areas of high technology in medicine vastly increase the cost of care and undermine the competence in its use.

6. Furthermore, medical technology and the system built upon it have now themselves become an increasingly important cause of disease and disability, both because of the inherent dangers of powerful diagnostic and therapeutic methods and because of their misuse by incompetent and venal personnel and institutions.

The technological power of modern medicine is awe-inspiring. So is its ability to do harm, both in the course of diagnosis and treatment. Diagnostic tests, in fact, may do considerably more harm than the illnesses they are supposed to detect or help diagnose. This is especially true when the tests are used for screening in otherwise healthy people, but it is also true for diagnostic tests for people who are clearly ill.

One of the most criticized forms of diagnostic testing is that of X rays. According to surveys by the U.S. Public Health Service in 1970, 129 million Americans (over 50 percent of the population) were given 210 million medical and dental X-ray examinations involving a total of 650 million films. That amounts to an average of over three X-ray films per year for every man, woman and child in the United States. It has been estimated that current annual radiation exposure from all medical sources results in as many as 13,500 serious disabilities and 7500 deaths from cancer.

Some diagnostic X rays are unquestionably of direct benefit to the people on whom they are performed, but many X-ray examinations could be avoided or at least deferred, and even the necessary ones are often done with insufficient safeguards against unnecessarily high levels of radiation.

The determination that an X-ray examination is unnecessary or deferrable for a sick person (like the determination, which we will explore in a moment, that a medication or an operation is unnecessary or deferrable) is difficult to prove in the individual case, and the evidence for excess exposure is largely statistical. One area, however, in which the statistics quite clearly point to dangerous overuse is in the use of X rays for screening for certain types of illness in people who have no symptoms or signs of the illnesses and no evidence of excess risk. An example is the use of mammography (a form of X ray of the breasts) which was at one time advocated for routine screening of women for early detection of breast cancer. Recent evidence suggests that the use of these X rays—with the possible exception of their use in women with high risk, such as those over the age of 50 or younger ones with a strong family history of breast cancer (and even this is arguable)—is likely to cause more cancer than is detected early enough to make a difference.

Even when the information to be provided by the X-ray examination may be necessary, there is often too much exposure. A study by the U.S. Bureau of Radiological Health found that in more than half of medical diagnostic X rays, the beam is larger than it needs to be for the desired information. Many X rays are taken by outmoded equipment that delivers a radiation dose unnecessarily high for the type of test being performed. In many states the equipment is not inspected regularly to determine whether it properly delivers the intended dose. Many X rays are taken by relatively untrained persons who may give an unnecessarily high dose either through poor technique or, more subtly, by producing poor-quality films so that more radiation exposure is received through repeat films. Even simple precautions are seldom used; for example, the use of a lead sheet to shield the parts of the body that need not show on the film, especially the reproductive organs. One estimate is that "with relatively little effort we could reduce medical exposure to radiation to one-tenth of its present value and at the same time enhance medical benefits."

Turning from the dangers of diagnosis to those of treatment, the two examples increasingly discussed are drugs and surgery. Each year approximately 300,000 Americans are hospitalized because of drug reactions, making this one of the ten leading causes of hospitalization in the United States. Some analysts have suggested that as many as 150,000 people may die each year as a result of drug reactions, although this figure is hotly disputed.

Undoubtedly, some use of dangerous drugs, despite their potential for adverse reactions, may be unavoidable, a reasonable and reasoned calculated risk recommended by the physician and accepted by the patient in the hope that the drug will help relieve some painful, seriously limiting or potentially dangerous problem. But too many of the prescriptions seem inappropriate, unnecessary, or both. American doctors write twice as many prescriptions per patient as do Scottish physicians. Since health-status data suggest that Scots are neither considerably sicker or healthier than Americans, a strong suspicion is raised that as many as half the prescriptions written by American physicians may be unnecessary.

The group of drugs that is most widely prescribed and the one that seems to cause the largest number of adverse reactions are the antibiotics. From 1967 to 1971 the population of the United States grew by about 5 percent; over the same period the number of antibiotic prescriptions filled grew 30 percent, some six times faster. In 1967 the average American was put on antibiotics once every two years; by 1971 the rate had climbed to nearly once a year. Yet there has been no significant change during the same period in the incidence of diseases for which antibiotic treatment would be helpful or in the types of antibiotics available. Indeed, only about once every five years does the average adult have an infection requiring antibiotics, and although the rate of infections in children may be higher, their numbers and their rates of illness are certainly not sufficient to account for the differences between the need for antibiotics and their use.

The dangers of unnecessary use of antibiotics, apart from the waste of resources that could be used productively in other ways, are twofold. The first is adverse reactions. Chloramphenicol, for example, is a powerful antibiotic useful for typhoid fever, Rocky Mountain spotted fever and other dangerous and uncommon infections. One of its side effects, however, is the production of aplastic anemia, which may often be fatal. Yet it has been estimated that one in every four prescriptions for the drug are for diseases in which it is known to be useless or for which there are safer alternatives.

The other danger is that of superinfections, the invasion of the body by another form of infectious agent to which the antibiotic has made the patient susceptible.

Another form of treatment that has been severely criticized for unnecessarily frequent use and for the incompetence of some of its practitioners is surgery. Of the approximately 18 million surgical operations in the United States in 1975, approximately 250,000 resulted in death during the surgery or during the post-operative period. In other words, roughly 1 out of every 75 operations ended in death for the patient. About four million of these operations were performed on an emergency basis; of these about 1 in 20 ended in death. Many of these patients, of course, were critically ill before their surgery and might well have died at about the same time if they had not had the operation. For many others, who lived, the operation was clearly a lifesaving procedure.

On the other hand, approximately 14 million of the 18 million operations performed in 1975 were elective, and among these elective operations approximately 1 in every 200 ended fatally. In these patients it was often the surgery or its complications that prematurely ended their lives. Many of these elective operations, even though not emergencies and therefore termed "elective," were necessary for the well-being of the patient, thus the risk was a reasonable one. However, in a large but unknown percentage of the operations, the surgery was unnecessary or deferrable—that is, the patient would have lived just as full a life, at worst with only slightly more disability or slightly less life expectancy, if the surgery had not been performed.

The reason the amount of "unnecessary surgery" is unknown is that it is often impossible to predict which patients will later get into serious trouble or whose disability will persist or get worse if they don't have the surgery as an elective procedure.

A patient, for example, with a diseased gallbladder not removed at the time it is discovered may have further warning symptoms prompting later removal, or may, except for manageable symptoms, have no further serious trouble. On the other hand, the patient may have serious complications or require much more dangerous emergency surgery if the gallbladder is not removed as an elective procedure.

One way of attempting to determine in advance which types of elective surgery might be postponed or deferred indefinitely is to get the opinion of a second surgeon. In one study in which a second opinion was compulsory for insurance coverage when surgery was recommended, in about 20 percent of cases the second surgeon felt that it could safely be postponed. When the surgery was postponed, a follow-up study on the patients showed that in the majority of cases it could be postponed for a year or longer. Even if the second surgeon is right in only half the instances of disagreement, these data suggest that some 10 percent of elective surgery may be safely deferrable, avoiding at least 10,000 unnecessary deaths and untold pain and disability associated with the surgery.

Furthermore, there are statistical studies within the United States—as well as international comparisons—which suggest that even this estimate of unnecessary surgery may be too low. In a study performed in Kansas in 1969, the rate of performance of six common operations varied as much as fourfold, depending on the number of surgeons and hospital beds per person in the area studied. In other studies, patients covered by prepaid health plans (in which surgeons are paid the same amount whether they operate or not) had about half as much surgery as those covered by Blue Shield (in which doctors received a fee for operations). In England and Wales there are only half as many operations per capita as in the United States; British surgeons are salaried and there are only half as many surgeons per capita in Britain as there are in the United States.

For certain types of elective surgery, the rate in comparable countries is even less than half the U.S. rate; in England and Wales, for example, the rate of hysterectomies is only 40 percent of that in the United States. Moreover, the number of board-certified surgeons in the United States is increasing rapidly. For many years, one-fourth of all U.S. medical graduates have entered training in surgery, and almost 3000 new fully trained surgeons are produced annually, bringing the total by 1975 to about one surgeon in every seven practicing physicians. The number of surgical procedures performed each year per 1000 population increases (about a 10-percent increase from 1970 to 1974 alone) to keep pace with the number of surgeons.

These data suggest that the criteria for surgery in the United States—even among those providing the second opinion—are related more to the availability of surgeons and the income they derive from performing surgery than to any absolute or even relative need of the patient for surgery.

Whether the surgery is necessary or deferrable or not, the chance of complications or of a fatal outcome rests in part on the competence of the surgeon, and there is considerable evidence that many do not perform at the highest level of quality. Some 30,000 physicians of the 82,000 who practice surgery full- or part-time in the United States (not counting the 12,000 doctors in surgical training who in principle at least perform surgery under some degree of expert supervision) have either never passed or never taken the examination for board certification of the American Board of Surgery. Furthermore, because of the relatively large number of doctors practicing surgery in the United States in proportion to its population, and because of their maldistribution, many surgeons perform only a few operations each week—this though most surgeons themselves believe that surgeons should average about ten operations a week in order to maintain their skills.

Unfortunately, the incompetent surgeon, it is generally agreed, is not the only type of incompetent physician in the United States. Approximately 16,000 licensed physicians, 5 percent of the country's doctors, are believed by the U.S. Federation of State Medical Boards—hardly a radical group or one given to making statements derogatory of physicians—to be unfit to practice medicine. Yet once a license to practice medicine is issued in the United States, it entitles a doctor to practice for the rest of his or her professional life without any evidence required of continued competence. An average of only 66 licenses a year *over the entire United States* are revoked by licensing boards, and those for the grossest of abuses such as overtly criminal acts or evidence of psychiatric illness or of drug abuse so flagrant that it can no longer be ignored.

Simultaneous with and apparently closely related to the increasing possibility of injury through the underuse, overuse or misuse of medical technology—and also, as we shall explore later in this chapter, to a rise in unrealistic expectations of the efficacy of medicine—is a rapid rise in the number of damage suits alleging malpractice on the part of physicians and medical institutions. The number decided in favor of the plaintiff is also rising—though apparently not at the same rate as the number of suits—and the size of the awards to the plaintiffs is rising, too. The lawyers who handle such suits argue that this is a mechanism not only to provide compensation to the injured patient and his family but also to punish incompetent physicians and institutions. Some see these suits as one of the few ways that the individual—or the society as a whole—has of controlling its physicians.

Doctors and hospitals argue, conversely, that the frequency and the size of malpractice awards often seem to correlate poorly with the level of technical competence; in fact, the more specialized physicians who handle the technically most difficult problems—such as orthopedists and anesthesiologists—seem to be at far greater risk of malpractice suits than those who deal with less dramatic problems—such as pediatricians or general practitioners. Furthermore, they note, large malpractice awards have been granted even when there was no way that the physician could reasonably be expected to have known or even suspected that what was done was dangerous.

There is some truth in this. Recent examples are the suits related to cases of retrolental fibroplasia caused by the use of pure oxygen for breathing by premature infants in the 1950s. At the time the injury was caused it was not known that pure oxygen would cause such disability; the oxygen was used as a lifesaving measure. But the statute of limitations on suits related to such injuries to children only begins when they reach age 21; therefore suits can be brought a generation later when the state of knowledge has markedly changed. Such suits obviously cannot be viewed as a mechanism for controlling current competence, except insofar as they remind the medical profession that failure to adequately evaluate drugs before they are prescribed can lead to unnecessary hazards for the patient.

The medical profession almost universally feels that the threat of malpractice suits leads to "defensive medicine"—the use of even more diagnostic tests, for example, which further drives up the cost of medical care and leads to increased discomfort and potential risk. Coupled with the fact that only a small percentage of the large premiums paid by physicians and hospitals for malpractice insurance finds its way into the hands of those who have suffered injury—most of it goes to the lawyers, on both sides, and to other costs of the litigation and insurance process—malpractice suits as a way of dealing with incompetence, or even as a way of compensating patients for their injuries at the hands of the medical-care system, seem particularly ineffective and self-defeating.

In sum, both the technology itself and some of society's defenses against it lead to an expanding cycle of further technology in an attempt to control that which we have. The system seems in many ways to be out of control.

7. The investment of human resources in the U.S. medical-care system is also massive—and the personnel structure of the system is authoritarian and hierarchical, dominated by physicians who are largely drawn from the intellectual and social elite, with other health workers having relatively little status, power, upward mobility or satisfaction.

Health care is not only a huge industry when measured by the amount of money and technology poured into it, it is also huge in terms of the number of people employed in it. As shown in Figure 13, almost five million people work in health care—some 5 percent of the employed population of the United States.

Of these health workers, approximately one-half—some two and a half million—are employed in providing what are called "nursing services," including registered nurses, licensed practical nurses, nurses' aides, orderlies and home health aides. About 375,000 (8 percent) are physicians, most with the M.D. degree, but also including a much smaller number with the degree of doctor of osteopathy, who in all states are licensed to do anything that a physician with an M.D. degree can do. The remainder are employed in approximately 100 other skilled and unskilled occupations, including such varied roles as ambulance attendants, laboratory technicians, pharmacists, receptionists, radiologic technicians, dieticians, secretaries, dental assistants and research scientists.

Over the panoply of facilities and people that is the U.S. medical-care system, the physician has reigned supreme. His or (rarely, but increasingly) her dominance over the U.S. health system has been derived, at least in part, from his authority over and dominance of his patients, a phenomenon which has existed since prehistoric times when the practice of medicine originated in magic and was a priestly art.

There are, of course, still elements of the priesthood in the physician's role, in how he sees himself and how he is viewed by patients and coworkers alike. The authority of the physician today is still based both on the "authority of office" (that is, on the fact that he is a member of the guild), on the "authority of knowledge" (that is, on the assumption that he has special technical competence) and on the "authority of class" (that is, on the often vast social-class difference between him and other health workers or patients). Because the technical competence is more complex and more powerful than ever before, and because the income and prestige differences are huge and increasing, today more than ever his authority takes precedence over all others in the health field.

The physician guards the powers conferred on him, in part

FIGURE 13

Number of Health Workers in the United States, 1900–1974

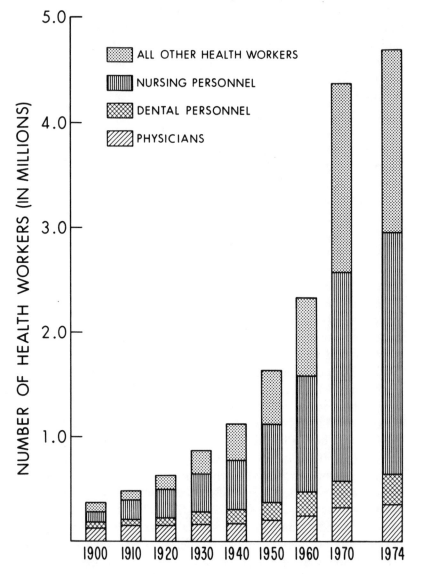

Prepared by the authors from data published by the National Center for Health Statistics.

by controlling the information made available to patients and to the general public, a control as rigid in its technological form as was the ancient guarding of priestly rituals. A fictionalized account of one physician's internship vividly conveys this withholding of information and its function:

> I didn't show her the X-rays; none of us ever showed parents the studies themselves. It was a kind of informal tradition that you were to interpret what the lab results revealed, not show the tests. The idea was not to make the parents nervous with technical details they were not prepared to understand. That it could also be a device to keep control, to keep the mystery—and patient respect—alive and working, had not occurred to me then.

But there are even larger issues at stake than the mystification of the individual patient and family. The physician is now in a position to control vast resources—resources for medical-care services, for medical education and for research. In an age when billions of dollars are spent at the bidding of technologists and technocrats and when the vast majority of the people in every society possesses insufficient knowledge and information (as opposed to intelligence and judgment) on which to base sound decisions, physicians and other technocrats of medicine become extraordinarily powerful in the technological decision-making process.

Furthermore, the process itself becomes self-perpetuating, the technology becomes an end in itself, and the only ones who can discuss the technology with adequate understanding (who have the tools to deal with the issues) are those who control it. What should be a political decision, in its original sense—made with the good of the polity in view—often becomes a narrow technical decision made by those whose judgment must at least in part be colored by their view of what's in it for them.

Between the macrocosm of social policy and the microcosm of the doctor's office, the modern U.S. hospital has come more and more to resemble a modern industrial plant with its elaborate division of labor and the increasing alienation of the hospital worker. Most hospital workers remain at their entry-level jobs unless they acquire more formal training or other credentials even though they often learn skills on the job and perform tasks at a higher level.

The result is a rigid occupational hierarchy with an elaborate system of rank identifications such as uniforms and titles and an equally rigid social-class system. In 1970, 98 percent of U.S. physicians were white, 91 percent were male and predominantly from middle- and upper-middle-class families; while 92 percent of nurses were white, 98 percent were female and from predominantly middle- and lower-middle-class families. Of the total enrolled in training programs administered by hospitals in 1973–74, 86 percent of practical-nurse trainees were white and 96 percent were female; while 64 percent of nurse's-aide trainees were white and 87 percent were female, and 64 percent of orderly-trainees were white and 14 percent were female.

Thus it is clear that in general as income and power drop, the domination by white males ends and medical professions become overwhelmingly female and increasingly nonwhite. As one practical nurse described the hierarchy in the hospital where she worked, "You have to see this place as a giant bureaucracy. I'm at the bottom of it, or maybe the patients are, and there's not a lot an individual can do."

The physician is of course at the top of the medical-care structure, earns the most money, as is shown in Figure 14, and has the most power. As the figure shows, the income differentials between those at the top and those at the bottom have markedly increased over the past two decades.

The nurse is typically subordinate to both the physician and the hospital, and early in her training learns to play what one observer has called the "doctor-nurse game," the object of which is that the nurse "be bold, have initiative and be responsible for making significant recommendations, while at the same time [appearing] passive." She must "make her recommendations appear to be initiated by the physicians," taking care not to disturb the physician's narcissism or feelings of omnipotence.

FIGURE 14

Income of Selected Health Workers
1949–1970

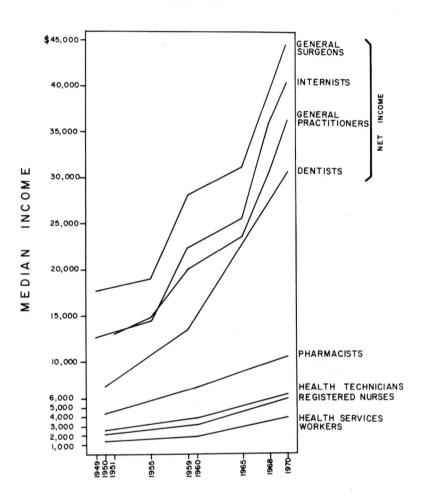

Reprinted from Vincente Navarro, *Medicine Under Capitalism* (New York: Prodist, 1976), p. 141. Used by permission.

The doctor's role vis-à-vis other health professionals and paraprofessionals is even more distant and authoritarian. In hospital settings those persons who are in continuous and intimate contact with patients are workers with the lowest status and least power in the institution. Eliot Friedson's description of the alienated industrial worker seems to fit the medical paraprofessional as well:

> Lacking identification with the prime goals of the organization, lacking an important voice in setting the formal level and direction of work, and performing work that has been so rationalized as to become mechanical and meaningless, a minute segment of an intricate mosaic of specialized activities that he is in no position to perceive or understand, the worker is alienated.

In spite of this alienation, more and more of the caring functions of medicine are left to the nurse's aides, the LPNs, the orderlies. Furthermore, since workers in the primarily female caring professionals of nursing and social work have been awakened to their low status by the women's movement, members of these professions have in significant numbers attempted to "move up" into traditionally male and therefore higher-status teaching or administrative roles, leaving the caring function increasingly to powerless paraprofessionals with still lower status.

Thus we may view the typical structure of a large medical institution as a pyramid with the usually white, male physician on top, his orders carried out by middle-level professionals who are generally women, and with the patients and the "dirty work" left to low-paid, frequently alienated, largely black female paraprofessionals at the bottom of the pyramid.

Although acceptance into medical school has shifted somewhat in recent years toward the female (24 percent of the entering class in 1975 compared to 6 percent 20 years earlier) and toward "minority" students (8 percent of the entering class in 1975), the more pronounced trend has been toward higher and higher intellectual requirements; the percentage of students with A averages in medical school has increased from 13 percent in 1965 to 44 percent in 1975. This, together with the rapid increase in medical school (and college) tuition—in one medical school now over $10,000 per year for four years—discriminates more and more against the socially and educationally disadvantaged. Yet, there is absolutely no evidence that intellectual attainment beyond a given level is necessary for technical proficiency or that intellectual attainment at any level is correlated with skill in providing humane medical care. Furthermore, the emphasis on grades, particularly in science courses, and the intense competition for the limited number of medical school places, has led to enormous anxieties among premedical students and a profound distortion of the undergraduate learning experiences.

Furthermore, once in medical school, the educational pattern is largely irrelevant—and actually seems to be inimical—to the practice of medicine, particularly of primary medical care. Much of the work in the preclinical sciences is based on the needs and desires of a "science" faculty and has little use meeting patients' needs. A very large percentage of the clinical work is done on (the word "on" is usually more appropriate than "with") hospitalized patients in large teaching hospitals. In most medical schools well over 50 percent of the teaching is done on "horizontal" rather than "vertical" patients. As Jack Geiger has commented, "It's like teaching forestry in a lumber yard." Moreover, while studies of how patients actually need and use medical care indicate that patients' needs lie largely outside the hospital, the teaching nevertheless concentrates on the small fraction of care that takes place not only in a hospital, but in the university medical center tertiary-care hospital.

Inappropriate intellectualization and academization of training occurs among other health workers as well. A recent report by the secretary of education of Massachusetts states that he finds absolutely no evidence that registered nurses who hold bachelor's degrees are any more competent in patient care than are those who have graduated from hospital-based schools, yet diploma nurses find it difficult to get jobs at comparable pay to baccalaureate nurses. Registered nurses with diplomas, the report stated, find themselves "squeezed" between the registered nurses with bachelor's degrees, on one hand, and the licensed practical nurses, who have lesser levels of technical skills and thus command far less salary, on the other. At all of these levels, nurses, like other health workers, are judged more by how academic their training was and by their degrees and licenses than by what they can actually do for the patient.

New categories of personnel are constantly being added to the system, both in response to the demands of technology and to the demands of patient care. One response over the past ten years to the shortage and inappropriate use of health personnel has been the development of physician's assistant programs. The effort has been highly publicized, but the number of new workers trained is still quite small.

The term "physician's assistant" includes a range of health workers—variously called physician's associates, MEDEX (for "medical extenders"), clinical associations, child-health associates and others. "Assistant to the primary-care physician," for example, is a generic term used for an assistant who performs certain specified tasks under the direction and supervision of a physician in a number of settings, from a physician's office to a hospital. The assistant has a wide range of duties which include taking patients' case histories, performing physical examinations, drawing blood samples, giving intravenous injections and infusions, providing immunizations, suturing and caring for wounds, and other specific tasks usually performed by doctors.

Programs to train PAs (the abbreviation is in part a way of avoiding the problem of whether they should be called "assistants" or "associates") were begun in the mid-1960s at a time when the Vietnam War was annually producing thousands of military medical corpsmen whose knowledge and experience were being lost to the civilian world after their discharge. Because the PA concept was originally seen as a way to utilize those trained in the military medical corps and at the same time provide needed medical manpower, the new medical professionals were expected to be predominantly male. The nursing profession, not unreasonably, saw the development as yet another device of the medical establishment to undercut the predominantly female nursing profession, and in response the new professional role of "nurse practitioner" has been developed.

Since the first PA program at Duke University in 1965, some 4000 students have graduated from the roughly 60 training programs now accredited by the AMA. The programs, which now graduate about 1300 PAs a year, vary enormously in their requirements and even in the length of the program. Some 40 states have enacted legislation governing the use of PAs.

Severe problems have developed. There are conflicts between PA and nurse-practitioner programs in determining status, hierarchy and which training programs will receive how much money from the federal government. Although most PAs are trained in primary care, some are already reflecting the specialization of the medical profession; they are being trained in such diverse medical specialties as anesthesiology, pathology, surgery, obstetrics and orthopedics, and in these roles the PAs are adding to the specialization within medicine rather than providing additional primary care.

And, of course, for the PA, as for the nurse practitioner, the nurse, the nurse's aide and other health workers, there is usually almost no chance to become a physician. The only pathway to advancement is through administration, supervision and teaching, with the result that the most skilled health workers either feel trapped and frustrated in their subsidiary roles or are forced to move further and further away from direct patient care.

Another, perhaps even more basic, criticism is that PAs and nurse practitioners may become the physicians for the poor while the rich are able to purchase and demand care by "real" doctors. While this criticism is still for the most part more theoretical than real, the danger in an unregulated, fee-for-service system certainly exists. The issue is how the medical-care system chooses to use these new workers—as part of an effort to bring greater equity to the system, or to further stratify the already highly stratified provision of health care.

Up to this point PAs are not changing the nature of American medicine but rather shoring up its current organization and priorities. Nationally, 77 percent of PA graduates are absorbed into private practices. The physicians who add PAs to their practice often charge their regular fees for a visit conducted entirely or largely by a PA, and pocket the difference between the PA's salary (from $7500 to $22,500 a year, relatively modest compared to a doctor's income) and the fee charged.

In short, these new health roles act to further the physician's control of the health-care system.

There are some areas, however, in which the physician's dominance of the medical-care system is being effectively threatened. The increasing size, complexity and corporate structure of the hospital give its professional managers new power over the workshop in which a large share of the physician's income is generated. The increasing cost of medical care and its major financing through insurance companies and tax levy funds give regulators and claims examiners new power over the physician's income and therefore over his pattern of practice.

The response of many physicians is to join together in what they view as—and sometimes call—"physician's unions." Strikes have been threatened, and over some issues, such as malpractice insurance rates, have even been partially carried out in some areas. While some physicians question the "ethics" of such actions—which, to be effective, will leave patients without a source of continuing or even emergency care—it seems likely that when the provocation is seen as large enough a significant percentage of physicians will be willing to use methods traditionally identified with the working class.

Some critics see unionization of physicians as a step forward, a breaking down of some of the elitist pretensions of the physician, even as a "proletarianization" of physicians. One major difference, of course, is that the threat to withhold services is often the only significant leverage available to workers wishing to improve their wages or working conditions, while most doctors already have other powerful resources and methods for control and change at their disposal. Another is that most workers are economically damaged by even a short strike, while most doctors can afford to strike for a prolonged period either because of their accumulated wealth or their expectation of future large incomes.

Others therefore fear that the elitist attitudes will not change but simply be further expressed through the power of organized deprivation of services, a deprivation which will become the ultimate weapon in the hands of an already powerful group.

8. The U.S. health- and medical-care system, while fostering high expectations of the efficacy of medical care and expanding its involvement in and control over more and more aspects of people's lives, is increasingly seen as depersonalized and uncaring.

Over the past 30 years there has been a marked change in the expectations of the public toward health and toward health care and medical care. These expectations take a variety of forms. First, there is the rising expectation that one will avoid dying at least until one's sixties and, particularly, that one will avoid dying of infectious desease. A half-century ago death at an early age from infectious disease was not uncommon. Today the occasional death from pneumonia or other infection in a young person and the occasional outbreak of infectious disease which kills a group of people are unexpected and are greeted with outrage. The feeling in such cases is that the medical-care system (for the individual patient) or the health-care system (in the case of an outbreak) has somehow not done its job.

Much higher numbers of deaths are tolerated, even somehow expected, when the cause is an accident (an airplane accident or major fire), and even more so when the cause of death is seen as a "natural phenomenon" such as an earthquake or a flash flood. Furthermore, "preventable" deaths from technology (*e.g.,* automobiles and war) seem somehow more acceptable than "preventable" deaths from "illness." The result is a tendency to blame the system for deaths that would at other times have been accepted as a part of nature or an act of God.

Another type of rising expectation is that of limitation of disability because of advances in medical treatment. Popular stories of open-heart surgery, of transplantation of kidneys and other organs, and of magical prostheses have made it hard to accept that any illness should still lead to long-term or permanent disability. The idea that it must be some kind of error of omission or commission that caused the disability makes it much harder to accept and to cope successfully with the disability. When such disabilities were accepted as a part of the natural vicissitudes of life, a matter of chance or of a malevolent and capricious God, one could rail, but it was clear that nothing effective could be done. Now one has something much more concrete to blame if treatment does not turn out well; it must be someone's fault.

These rises in expectations are, of course, part of the basis for the explosive increase in the number of malpractice suits and the size of the awards. If the cause of the disability is an act of omission or commission on the part of the health- or medical-care system, then someone in the system should be made to pay for it. On the one hand, the suit is seen as punitive; "pay" is seen in the retributive and controlling as well as the distributive sense. On the other hand, the malpractice suit is used for reimbursement or compensation. Outside of Workmen's Compensation, few vehicles for socially supplied compensation and support for injury or illness exist; there are few forms of "no fault" insurance which make compensation available to victims whether the disability was the result of a failure in the prevention or treatment system or not.

Paradoxically, while expectations have risen dramatically in the technical areas of medical practice, they have fallen in other areas. Very few people these days expect that their physicians will make home visits, or even that they will take the time for full discussion of symptoms, diagnosis or treatment. But while they don't expect such care, patients nevertheless often become disaffected when these negative expectations are proved correct. Home visits, for example, have declined from 10 percent of all ambulatory physician visits in 1958 to 1 percent in 1974. And the complaint is frequently heard that doctors don't have enough time to respond to the other-than-technological needs of their patients.

Since it is difficult to measure the adequacy of response to the patient as a human being who is anxious and needs help, reassurance or education, rather than as a set of complex organ systems which need "fixing," most of the evidence for inadequate responsiveness must be anecdotal rather than statistical. There are stories in abundance of the gynecologist who doesn't warm the speculum; of the pediatrician who doesn't take the time to explain to the child what the procedure will be like; of the professor who brings the medical students in without regard for the patient's wishes; of the researcher who uses the dependency of the patient as a lever to get consent for the research, or doesn't bother to get properly informed consent at all; and of doctors who talk to each other, oblivious of the patient's presence, in terms that the patient is expected not to understand but often understands only too well.

As large amounts of primary medical care are practiced in emergency rooms, medical care is frequently carried on by doctors who expect—or even hope—never to see the patient again, and who behave accordingly. There are also complaints about office hours that are often established for the convenience of the doctor or other personnel with little regard for the needs of patients. Complaints are particularly prevalent among hospitalized patients: the unappetizing food served cold; the unresponded-to bell; the unanswered questions; the lack of personal introduction or even of formal identification of people who come into the room to play a part in the diagnostic or treatment procedures; the long waits in cold X-ray departments; the placement of inappropriate patients together in the same room; transfer to other floors to suit the convenience of doctors or of "educational" or institutional needs, taking the patient away from familiar nurses or friendships with other patients.

The tendency of health workers to view patients as a series of symptoms or mechanical problems is vividly described by Duff and Hollingshead in their study of a large East Coast teaching hospital:

> No ward patient thought there was a physician to whom he could talk about his fears of hospitalization, illness or treatment. . . .Visitors . . . who watched the desperate behavior of the patients and listened to their conversations were swept along in the current of intense, sincere, emotionally painful yet awe-inspiring and tragic efforts of the sick to cope with their fears. These efforts were almost entirely ignored by the physicians, nurses and other members of the hospital staff.

In short, the patient is often forgotten in the effort to deal with the disease or in the effort to provide for the convenience of the practitioners or the institution.

A particular kind of depersonalization concerns patients with a set of cultural beliefs that are not shared or understood by the health worker. These often lead not only to what appears to the patient to be unfeeling care but to failure in diagnosis and treatment as well.

A set of well-documented examples concerns patients who have come to the United States from Puerto Rico. Many of these patients classify illnesses, medicines and foods according to an etiological and therapeutic system derived from the ancient Hippocratic humoral theory of disease. The theory states that health is manifested by a moderately wet, moderately warm body, a state of balance among four humors; and that illness, which causes the body to become excessively dry or wet, hot or cold or a combination of these states, is caused by a humoral imbalance. Food, herbs and medications are classified as wet or dry, hot or cold, and are used therapeutically to restore the body's balance. Thus, a "cold" disease, such as arthritis, is treated by administering "hot" medication, and a "hot" disease, such as diarrhea, by "cold" medications and foods. Fruit juices, for example, are considered "cold" and may not be an acceptable treatment to a Puerto Rican patient when he or she has a common cold, a "cold" disease; this may be true even when the physician prescribes the fruit juice as a means of potassium supplement for the patient on a diuretic, and the patient's reluctance to follow the advice may lead to complications of potassium depletion. Pregnant women may be reluctant to take iron supplements or vitamins, which are considered "hot," because they believe that "hot" foods and medications will cause the baby to be born with a rash.

Many Puerto Rican families also have a profound belief in spiritism, in the existence and specific influence of spirits on people's lives. Physical disabilities such as headaches, stomach pains, blindness, learning disorders in children and even heart attacks may be ascribed to the spirits. Patients with symptoms of physical illness frequently seek help from physicians or other health workers and, finding no solution, turn to a medium to exorcize the spirit causing the problem.

While it is extremely difficult to estimate what proportion of Puerto Rican families share a belief in this folk health system, the numbers are sufficiently large that awareness of the belief system and an ability to work within it are essential for health workers working with Puerto Rican patients. Unfortunately, far too often the health worker is either ignorant of the medical tradition or dismisses it as irrelevant and unscientific. Similar ignorance of or lack of sensitivity to patient's beliefs is often found among health workers who work with the Navaho or other native Americans or with immigrants whose roots lie in Oriental cultures. If a technique is held to be "unscientific" in the eyes of the health worker, it will often be ridiculed or even arbitrarily denied to the patient.

An extreme example of depersonalization, almost a caricature of modern medical practice, involves the use of television for remote-control interviews, examination and treatment. Michael Crichton in his book *Five Patients* has described the use of this technique by doctors of the Massachusetts General Hospital as part of the provision of medical services to Boston's

Logan Airport. With the aid of a nurse, two television cameras, a TV screen and a large instrument console, a 56-year-old passenger suffering from chest pain is interviewed and examined by a physician two and a half miles away. The physician is later quoted as saying that "talking by closed-circuit TV is really very little different from direct, personal interviews."

In addition, the patient's medical history can be taken by a computer and transmitted immediately to the physician. The Massachusetts General–Logan Airport computer program is actually a rather simple model; more complex programs for taking a computerized medical history already exist and will surely be used more extensively in the future. The development is not necessarily a bad one, since if properly applied as an adjunct to the caring health worker it can help prevent lapses in history-taking or in diagnosis which lead to incorrect treatment. But it is reasonable to predict, with the current structure of the medical-care system, that the technique will become an end in itself rather than a subordinate means and will lead to further dehumanization.

Even more disturbing than the lack of sensitivity to the special needs of people from different cultural traditions and the depersonalization—sins of omission, if you will—are the sins of commission, the biases in diagnosis and treatment, which are built into medical practice. Bias on the basis of social class, for example, has been demonstrated in a wide variety of studies. Patients with similar types of psychiatric illness have been shown to be treated differently—electric shock more likely for the poor, psychotherapy more likely for the affluent—and by different doctors—doctors-in-training more likely for the poor, fully trained and experienced doctors for the rich.

Patients from different social classes are also known to be handled differently in emergency rooms, with decisions often based on the way the unaccompanied patient is dressed when he or she is brought in; much more resuscitative effort is likely to be expended on the man brought in in a suit and tie than on one with dirty, disheveled clothes. Even when there is time to reflect and examine the biases, as in decisions for who would receive hemodialysis when resources were in short supply, the decisions clearly have class biases built into them.

Ironically, while the medical-care system is increasingly criticized for its dehumanizing reliance on technology and its insensitivity to patients' needs and feelings, it is simultaneously enveloping many aspects of people's daily lives. Aspects of daily life that were once managed by the individual, the nuclear family, the extended family, friends, neighbors or others in the community have over the past 30 years been increasingly "expropriated," to use Ivan Illich's term, by the health establishment or have been handed over to health professionals by bewildered lay people. Questions about breast-feeding, concern about a child's bed-wetting, ways to encourage an overweight teen-ager to diet were once matters to be discussed with older, more experienced family members. Methods of parenting, problems with sex or the anguish of death and dying were either kept inside the immediate family or shared with a few intimate friends. These concerns are often now treated as medical problems and brought to medical professionals, with a consequent loss of the feeling of being able to cope and loss of feeling of control over aspects of daily life by individuals and by families.

In addition to the medical system's outreach into the realm of what were formerly considered "personal" problems, it has also reached into the realm of what were once seen as legal or moral issues. Medical expropriation of the area of alcholism, drug abuse, child abuse or even teen-age vandalism has in recent years caused the medical-care system increasingly to become an institution of social control. Measures of control which a generation ago were the responsibility of the family, the police, the judge or the clergyman are now the responsibility of the health-care system.

While medicalization of behavior the society deems deviant has been accompanied by and to some extent caused by the decriminalization of that behavior, at least in the middle class, the question remains whether the medicalization is any less repressive, any less punitive than former sanctions. Is medicalization simply a "civilized" society's way of "managing" unpleasant behavior within society?

Again, the response of the individual is often to feel increasingly powerless, less able to "cope."

Ivan Illich has termed this undermining of social organization and of people's confidence in their own ability to cope "social iatrogenesis." To quote Illich:

> Social iatrogenesis is at work when health care is turned into a standardized item, a staple; when all suffering is "hospitalized" and homes become inhospitable to birth, sickness, and death; when the language in which people could experience their bodies is turned into bureaucratic gobbledegook; or when suffering, mourning, and healing outside the patient role are labeled a form of deviance. . . . Social iatrogenesis [is that phenomenon] in which the environment is deprived of those conditions that endow individuals, families, and neighborhoods with control over their own internal states and over their milieu.

But a central question of our age must be whether we can hope to return to "individuals, families, and neighborhoods . . . control over their own internal states" and over their own reality when we have such easily accessible methods to alter our perception of reality. In Irving Zola's words, ". . . we have drugs for nearly every mood; to help us sleep or keep us awake; to enhance our appetite or decrease it; to tone down our energy level or to increase it; to relieve our depression or stimulate our interest." Can we hope to compete with such an armamentarium? It is in part this very array of tools which gives the medical profession its power and makes others in the environment seem impotent in comparison.

Yet another crucial component of the pervasive power of the medical-care system in American society and in many other societies is mystification—both of the individual patient and of the society as a whole. Once such normal events of the human life cycle as breast-feeding, sexual activities, parenting and dying are medicalized, the potential for mass mystification by medical-care professionals is endless.

While mystification has taken on new dimensions due to the medicalization of society and to the technological revolution, it is by no means new to the practice of medicine. When doctors were indistinguishable from priests—as in ancient Greece or among Navaho medicine men—much of their power to heal lay in the faith of people in that power. That faith was in part dependent on their possession, and careful guarding, of a body of secrets and of access to the gods that only they possessed. Their exclusive possession of these secrets also, of course, maintained their own status and increased their power, prestige and earnings.

It is almost surely true that a portion of the healing process remains rooted in the patient's faith in the health worker, though exactly how much and for what types of illness and for what kinds of patients and health workers is far from clear. The fact is that the tools now available to the health worker have much more potential for either good or harm than did appeals to the gods. Thus traditional mystification has in large part remained even though the power of the physician to understand the biochemical and physiological roots of illness and to affect its course has changed dramatically.

The justification expressed for continued mystification takes several forms. One, where placebo therapy of some sort (the "sugar pill" in a variety of sizes and colors) is being used, is similar to the classic justification: If the patient knew the truth, faith would be lost and the treatment wouldn't work. Another justification is that the explanation would be too complex or technical and the physician has insufficient time for a presentation that could be truly comprehended and whose implications would be thoroughly understood by the patient or the patient's family. Yet another argument for mystification is that a full explanation would only cause the patient unnecessary anxiety or anguish. This argument is strengthened for physicians by patients who tell them explicitly that they "don't want to know" or who cut off attempts at the explanation of alternatives by asking the doctor to "tell me what to do."

While all of these arguments certainly have elements of validity, their frequent use is brought under suspicion by that other effect of mystification which has continued through the millennia—the strengthening of the status, power and rewards of the doctor.

9. The U.S. medical-care system also helps to produce similar problems in other countries, importing resources from countries that can ill afford to lose them and exporting inappropriate services and models to countries that can ill afford to invest in them and are often crippled by them.

Finally, not content with the problems created in our own country, the U.S. health-care and medical-care system creates problems in other countries. It drains off able and highly trained manpower from poorer countries; it drains off financial resources from the health-care sectors of other countries in the form of profits for U.S. manufacturers of drugs, medical equipment and other products; it provides models, based on those in the United States, that are clearly inappropriate for the countries to which they are transplanted; and even when it provides foreign "aid" in health areas, the aid is often tied directly or indirectly to U.S. products, U.S. consultants, and U.S. models.

The problem of the medical "brain drain" to the United States from poorer countries, particularly of physicians, but also of nurses and other skilled health workers, has been widely publicized in recent years. At the beginning of 1974 there were over 70,000 physicians in the United States who had graduated from foreign medical schools; approximately 60,000 of them were providing patient care, roughly one-fifth of the total physicians in the United States providing care. In 1973, 45 percent of the new medical licenses issued in the United States were issued to graduates of schools outside the United States.

Although the majority of these graduates ostensibly come to the United States for specialty training with the intention of returning to their homelands with added skills, most of them never make it back. Of foreign medical graduates identified in the AMA registry in 1963, 84 percent could still be identified as residing in the United States in 1971, and some of the remaining 16 percent could almost certainly be presumed to have retired, died or gone elsewhere than back to the country which had provided their medical training. Even if one limits the search to the foreign graduates who were interns or residents in 1963, 74 percent were still in the United States eight years later.

Most of the countries from which these doctors came can ill afford to lose them. True, a small percentage of these graduates are American citizens who, unable to gain admission to U.S. medical schools, went abroad for their medical education. But even for those students the country in which they were trained has almost certainly invested more resources—in one form or another—in their education than is compensated by their tuition payments. For the students who are nationals of the countries in which they are trained, the loss is both in human resources and in educational resources.

The impact of the loss of these physicians on the "donor" countries has only begun to be explored. One country that has explored the consequences in some depth is Iran, no longer one of the world's poorest countries, but still one with severe physician shortages. It is one of the four countries highest on the list of numbers of physicians emigrating to the United States. In 1972 there were at least 2000 Iranian physicians practicing in the United States, more than one-fifth of the total number of Iranian physicians practicing in Iran in the same year. In Iran's countryside, where more than 60 percent of its population lives, there are areas with as few as one physician per 100,000 population. Iran has responded, of course, by raiding ("recruiting campaigns" they are called) countries poorer than Iran, such as India, the Philippines and Pakistan.

In certain categories of work, particularly those with the lowest pay and the longest hours, and in certain hospitals, particularly those avoided by U.S. graduates, the percentage of FMGs (foreign medical graduates) is extremely high. At the beginning of 1972, for example, 33 percent of the interns and residents in the United States were FMGs. There is little evidence that the technological competence of the FMGs is—on the average, with some individual exceptions—less than that of U.S.-trained physicians; the main problem produced in the United States is usually not technical incompetence but rather the inability of some of the FMGs to communicate effectively with patients.

Again there are exceptions. A physician trained in Latin America may be better able to communicate with a Hispanic patient in the South Bronx than a physician raised and trained in almost any part of the United States. But the bringing of such a patient and such a doctor together is usually simply a matter of chance rather than a planned attempt to meet patient needs. Much more often there is a cultural and linguistic mismatch between doctor and patient, and at times a kind of veterinary medicine is practiced, based on physical examination rather than on a careful history of symptoms and disabilities, and on pills and physical treatment rather than on reassurance and advice.

There are yet other negative consequences to the United States of our use of personnel trained in other countries. As a result of the availability of this source of immigrant labor, the United States has become dependent on them and changes in medical education and in medical practice which would lessen the need for FMGs remain unaccomplished. When an attempt finally was made, by the enactment of legislation in 1976, to limit the entry of foreign nationals trained outside the United States and to ensure that those who do enter for training return to their homelands, its implementation was in part postponed because of the severe disruption in U.S. medical care the exclusion of FMGs would cause.

Nothing in this discussion, of course, should be taken as an argument against the freedom of all people—not only health workers—to leave their homelands in the face of political repression. Nor should it be taken as an argument against the responsibility of the United States to admit refugees from oppression. The issue of admitting political refugees clearly takes precedence over the problems created by their admission. But only rarely is political repression the cause of leaving.

Profit-making by U.S. companies in poor countries takes a number of forms, and some of the consequences are even more destructive than the withdrawal of the profits. The sale of drugs in developing countries by multinational corporations, many of them headquartered in the United States, is one of the best examples.

Not that the removal of resources through profits on drugs is not serious enough. While some cases of actual fraud have been uncovered, U.S.-based companies do not need to use fraudulent practices in order to remove large amounts of resources from the dependent country. As noted earlier, annual domestic sales for U.S.-based drug companies rose from $1.5 billion in 1955 to $6.5 billion in 1974, a fourfold increase in two decades. But foreign sales leaped from $0.4 billion in 1955 to $5 billion in 1974, a tenfold increase, and it has been predicted that foreign sales will soon exceed domestic sales.

Profits on the foreign sales can be enormous. In 1974 one U.S. company, for example, had a net profit from U.S. operations of 16.7 percent of its net worth; the comparative figure from foreign operations was 39.6 percent! Another made a net profit of 21.1 percent on domestic operations, and 34.1 percent on foreign operations.

But there are other consequences of drug sales in developing countries that are of greater immediate concern. Advertising practices for the same drug by a multinational company are often quite different in the United States, where advertising is controlled by the Food and Drug Administration, from their advertising in a developing country. Not only are drugs pushed in poor countries for use by patients with diseases for which these drugs cannot legally be advertised in the United States, but warnings required here pertaining to adverse reactions are often omitted in poor countries.

A particularly dangerous example is chloramphenicol, an

extremely powerful antibiotic which, as we have already discussed, can also cause fatal anemias. In the United States in 1973 chloramphenicol was advertised by its manufacturer for use only in patients with acute typhoid fever and other serious infections caused by strains of bacteria specifically susceptible to the drug; it was advertised in Mexico for tonsillitis, ear infections, urinary-tract infections and a wide range of other illnesses. In the United States, the manufacturer was required to list a long series of contraindications and warnings of adverse reactions, including the fact that the anemia which might be produced was potentially fatal; in Central America and Argentina not a single contraindication or adverse reaction was listed.

The failure to publicize the risks was so obvious and so dangerous that the Pan American Health Organization (the regional office for the Americas of the World Health Organization), in an unprecedented action, transmitted warnings against the unjustified use of chloramphenicol to all Latin American countries. The warning, of course, had far less impact than the drug company's advertising.

Another example is the marketing of the drug indomethacin. It is an extremely powerful weapon against the pain of arthritis, but can cause ulcers of the gastrointestinal tract, toxic hepatitis and other serious and potentially fatal complications. Furthermore, there is a relatively safe, inexpensive and effective drug for arthritis pain—aspirin. In the United States, the manufacturer is required to limit its recommendation for use of indomethacin to severe forms of arthritis; in Brazil, Ecuador, Colombia and Central America it is advertized for "lumbago" and a range of other ailments.

Still another striking example of destruction of health through profit-making is the effort by manufacturers of infant formulas, through various marketing techniques, to persuade mothers in poor countries to abandon their own nutritionally preferable breast milk and buy instead powdered formula or condensed milk. This, although the risk of bottle-feeding for those without pure water and refrigeration is enormous, and is believed to be one of the major causes of high infant mortality.

The problem has been exacerbated in recent years because

U.S. and European manufacturers of infant formulas, facing a decline in birth rates at home, have been stepping up their efforts to sell their products in developing countries, where birth rates remain high. The manufacturers use a variety of techniques to reach their target groups: performances, clowns, billboards and other advertisements, or publications—many of them aimed specifically at low-income people. According to a study done by Cornell University nutritionists, the "advertisements imply that nice people with nice homes who want nice babies, bottle-feed their babies."

Perhaps most pernicious, however, is the export of health and medical models which, however counterproductive for health in the United States, are even more inappropriate for less affluent countries. These inappropriate models include the use of high technology and highly trained professionals in countries whose urgent health-care needs would be far better met by improved sanitation, adequate nutrition and accessible primary care. The building of huge hospitals and medical centers with the latest technology in countries which cannot staff them and which desperately need basic preventive medicine and primary care in the villages where most of their people live may represent a great loss to their health care. When these models are tied to foreign aid by the United States, the seduction of "modern" methods may be too strong for even dedicated health officials in developing countries to resist.

The Rockefeller Foundation, particularly earlier in this century, and the United States Agency for International Development (AID) now are examples of this kind of effort. In the Philippines, the Foundation sent a hospital ship to bring the "benefits of civilization" to rebellious tribesmen. As George Vincent, the Foundation president, described the effort, "Dispensaries and physicians have of late been peacefully penetrating areas of the Philippine Islands and demonstrating the fact that for purposes of placating primitive and suspicious peoples medicine has some advantages over machine guns." Statements by officials of AID and other current foreign aid agencies are usually less blunt, and the methods more subtle, but the principles remain the same.

In short, the U.S. health- and medical-care system, wasteful and dangerous as it is for the people of the United States, also helps drain the resources, changes the priorities, and further undermines the health of the people of many of the poor countries of the world.

Part 2

Health Care and Medical Care in Other Countries

INTRODUCTION

There are pivotal questions whose answers help determine the structure of a society's health-care and medical-care system: What constitutes a healthy life and what constitutes disability? What human problems does one society elect to institutionalize and another society elect to care for in the community? What aspects of health care are viewed as individual or familial or private responsibility and what aspects are viewed as collective or societal or public responsibility? Whom shall medicine serve, and at what cost?

The answers to these questions are rooted in the history, the politics, the economics and the culture of each society. Furthermore, the structural forms created to meet societal needs—centralized or decentralized, corporate or individual, publicly controlled or privately controlled—are also products of the history, the politics, the economics and the culture of a society. Thus, to begin to understand the present, it is essential to attempt to tease apart the major threads which have been woven into the health-care institutions of a society, to discover the particular set of suppositions under which a society makes its decisions in one of its most emotionally charged areas—that of health and illness.

But the health-care and medical-care system of a society not only reflects that society's past, it also helps to mold its present and its future. Health care and medical care have frequently been used in other societies to further broaden social goals, as a cutting edge for social change. Therefore, having explored some of the current problems of health care and medical care in the United States, we turn now to an exploration of the systems in other countries, in the belief that a description and analysis of the ways in which health care and medical care have been structured in other societies can help us to think beyond the set of assumptions that usually constrain the analysis of our system.

For this purpose we have intentionally chosen countries with systems quite different from our own: Sweden with its mixture of public and private, centralized and decentralized health and medical care; Great Britain with its National Health Service based around the general practitioner; the Soviet Union with its highly centralized, comprehensive system; and China with its emphasis on local participation. All represent efforts to evolve ways of providing health care and medical care; each approach stems from the history and culture of that society; each demonstrates an attempt to meet some of the basic needs of the people. While, as noted earlier, it would be impossible to attempt direct transplantation of the methods these societies have used to a country whose system has quite different historical roots and is embedded in a quite different set of political, economic, social and cultural characteristics, their methods may nevertheless give us insights into ways we might approach our own problems.

First of all, analysis of the experience of these four countries demonstrates that while their responses have been quite different, each of them has been plagued by a number of problems held in common. Each country has been characterized by an unequal distribution of resources—in the society in general and in medical care in particular—and each of them, in its own way, has used the medical-care system to further a more equitable distribution of resources. Each country has had particular difficulty in providing accessible medical care in rural areas, and each in its own way has attempted to pull or push doctors and other health workers into the countryside. Each country has had significant problems with its doctors—generally an elitist group who are increasingly wedded to technology, and whose dominance over other health workers and over society is heightened by their control of a powerful technology—and each in its own way has attempted to seduce or mandate its doctors into greater social responsibility. Each country has faced a rapidly expanding technology and rapidly escalating costs, and each in its own way has attempted to bring the technology under social control. And each country—with the exception of China—has had great difficulty in integrating community participation into the provision of health care and medical care and, perhaps significantly, has made little progress in solving this problem.

For each of the four countries we start with a brief description of the setting, and then, to give a flavor of a central aspect of the health-care and medical-care system, we provide a brief description of one of its features which seems most characteristic and noteworthy. Following this, in each case, we turn to an overview of the historical roots of the current system. Finally, we describe the remaining relevant aspects of the medical-care system and attempt to summarize its strengths and remaining problems. Overall, our descriptions are selective rather than exhaustive, and reflect our view of the elements of health care, and particularly of medical care, in each country which are of greatest relevance to our own.

A word of caution must be raised before we begin: The same words often have different meanings in different societies, and different words are often used to describe the same phenomena. Moreover, as we have already discussed, statistics may be collected and used in quite different ways. Finally, internal differences may be great and, to a certain extent, defy generalization. Nonetheless, each of the countries—including our own—has patterns which transcend intranational variations and which are different enough that transnational comparisons appear to be valid and illuminating.

SWEDEN—
Planned
Pluralism

Sweden, a society with one of the world's highest standards of living and a "mixed economy," has attempted to provide medical care through "planned pluralism," a complex mixture of central and local, public and private services.

The Setting

Comparisons between Sweden and the United States are often questioned because of Sweden's relatively small size and its relative "homogeneity." Both qualifications are apt. Sweden's eight million people, equal to the population of New York City, live in a territory the size of California. The only serious challenge to its homogeneity lies in its immigrants ("foreign subjects") who comprise 5 percent of the population, do some of the most menial jobs and earn some of the lowest incomes, and who represent a discordant note in Swedish society which many Americans would recognize. But Sweden's immigrants are the recipients of large amounts of social services and of other efforts for their welfare, and stand out primarily because of the relatively high level of material wealth among the majority of Swedish people.

Despite these important differences, there are great similarities to the United States, similarities that make Sweden, in these characteristics at least, far more like the United States than any of the other countries discussed in this book. For example: Sweden is one of the few countries of the world which matches or exceeds the United States in level of technology, in gross national product per person, and in level of urbanization; private owners in Sweden control about 90 percent of the means of production of capital and consumer products; Sweden's political forms—even in view of its figurehead monarchy and its parliamentary-ministerial type of government—are not very different than those of the United States; and the vast majority of its people—apparently an even higher percentage than in the United States—live lives characterized by material comfort and considerable leisure time.

Along with its similarity to the United States in some of its successes, Sweden has similarities in failure as well. Alienation and discontent are phenomena of increasing concern in Sweden. Rapid urbanization has led to abrupt discontinuities with Sweden's rural past, with a consequent sense for many of its people of loss of community and identity (especially what many feel to be a loss of the values and satisfactions of identity with the land and its forests and lakes), and a loss of a sense of purpose among many of its youth. The result is a characteristic longing by many for a more rural and more communal life and a different pattern of human relationships, as seems to be the case in most industrialized countries.

Sweden is of particular interest to us because the health of the people, by almost any statistical measure, is equal to or better than the health of the people of any other country. As we have seen, its infant mortality rate is the lowest and its maternal mortality and age-specific mortality rates among the lowest in the world. Among the industrialized countries it is one of the lowest in the rate of deaths from motor vehicle accidents and in the number of cigarettes smoked per adult in the population, although smoking is rapidly increasing, especially among women. It stands not quite so well in some other areas of health status—such as alcoholism, which is said to constitute a problem in 10 percent of the male population—but its health problems are small compared to its overall record.

Sweden's medical-care system—which of course is only one of the factors, and probably not the most important one, in its excellent health status—has features that are of interest to us for a number of other reasons: (1) It is a pluralistic system, which includes a mix of "public" and "private" ownership, more comparable to that of the United States in a number of its features than the more single-modal systems of the other countries discussed here; (2) it is an expensive system with, as in the United States, more than 8 percent of the GNP devoted to health services; (3) it is a decentralized system with significant amounts of local financing, and therefore of local control of services, through the county councils and public health boards in local communities; (4) it has placed great stress simultaneously both on health care and on the most technological aspects of medical care; and (5) despite its practical pluralism and determined decentralization, it is a regionalized system, with vigorous and apparently relatively successful attempts to avoid duplication of costly equipment and specialists within each region.

An Attempt to Regionalize Medical Care

A central point of Sweden's experience with medical care is that Sweden, perhaps more than any other nonsocialist country, has over the past 15 years attempted to regionalize its medical-care services. Based on its historic governmental involvement in medical services and on governmental decentralization to the county level, and spurred by the rapidly rising cost of medical care during the 1960s, Sweden has sought to develop a system which would include a graded hierarchy of services and an integrated structure for decision-making and fiscal management.

Toward this end, seven health regions have been established, each encompassing between 650,000 and 1.6 million people.

Each region includes up to six counties, most of which have between 200,000 and 400,000 people, and, in turn, each county contains several health districts whose populations range from 7,000 to 40,000 people. Within regions, health services are provided at each of the three levels—the region, the county, the district.

The first level of care is provided in district health centers which have from one to fifteen doctors, as well as other medical personnel. It has been estimated that district health centers could provide approximately 75 to 80 percent of all outpatient care including individual preventive health care—far more than they currently provide. Most of the physicians in district health centers are generalists, although the larger centers include specialists in, for example, pediatrics, obstetrics-gynecology, internal medicine and psychiatry.

For the second level of care, most counties contain two or three district or "normal" hospitals which serve several health districts encompassing 75,000 to 100,000 people. These are general hospitals, with fewer than 600 beds, which provide care for emergencies, such as accidents, heart attacks and strokes, and also provide general hospital care, such as general surgery, internal medicine, anesthesiology and diagnostic X rays. In addition, in each county there is one central county hospital with 500 to 1000 beds which provides both general hospital care for the immediately surrounding population and more specialized care for the county as a whole. For example, the county hospital not only provides care in internal medicine and surgery but also services in gynecology, ophthalmology and orthopedics, and sometimes in neurology, cardiology and urology.

A third level of care is available at the regional level. Seven regional hospital centers have now been established, one in each of the seven health regions; six of these centers serve simultaneously as medical-college teaching hospitals. "Superspeciality" services such as neurosurgery, plastic surgery, thoracic surgery and radiation therapy are available at this level. There is, of course, no extra cost to patients who are referred from county hospitals to regional hospitals; the counties pay the cost of care to the region.

A fourth, even more specialized level of care is available in a few regional hospitals where relatively rare special services—such as open-heart surgery, care of spinal injury patients, and transplantation work—are performed. Although there has been some resistance to regionalization, Sweden is making an extensive effort to avoid duplication of expensive services and to rationalize the most costly and prestigious sector of medical care, through the provision of services at the least costly level at which they can be effectively provided.

Historical Background

The establishment of a comprehensive health-care system in Sweden was facilitated by three historical factors: (1) Most hospitals in Sweden were traditionally owned and operated by the government; (2) the physicians who cared for the sick in the hospital were, from their initiation, largely salaried and essentially limited in their practice to the hospital; and (3) "Provident Societies" or "sickness funds" as a way of dealing with the costs of medical care and with the loss of income during illness have existed in Sweden since the time of the medieval guilds.

The forerunners of the current hospital system in Sweden were the *Helgeandshus* (domiciles for the sick and needy) and asylums. In the early sixteenth century Gustav Vasa, whose father had been among a group of noblemen and clergy killed by Christian II, organized a revolt which started in a mining district in central Sweden and spread throughout the country. After his election by the nobles in 1523 as king of Sweden, he devoted his 37-year reign to the reconstruction of the Swedish state. During the shift from Roman Catholicism to Lutheranism as the established church, the crown seized the properties of the Catholic church and also made annexations from the nobility, thus bringing some 60 percent of Swedish soil under state control.

As part of this "recall" of property, the state became the owner of the many social institutions and gradually took responsibility for their maintenance and operation. By the end of the seventeenth century the care of the chronically ill, then primarily in charity institutions for "incurables," and of those with contagious diseases was still carried out by the established church, but the city administration and the parish meeting had primary responsibility for them.

As early as 1663 a royal charter established the Collegium Medicum, the forerunner of the present National Board of Health and Welfare, and during the next century the sphere of responsibility of the Collegium was greatly extended. In 1774 it was commissioned by the government to "find out and publish what the so-called unknown diseases are that carry off, in part, the children of the peasantry" and was given responsibility for smallpox inoculations, for the supervision of the general care of the sick, and for the investigation and prevention of venereal diseases.

The first institution in Sweden expressly set up for treating acute illness and accidents—in contrast to the domiciliary function of its predecessors—was the mining hospital in Falun founded in 1639. The world-famous Seraphimer Hospital in Stockholm opened its doors in 1752. In 1756 a royal charter granted permission to the towns and rural districts to establish hospitals at their own expense but, increasingly, with some subsidization by the state. These hospitals, which became known as "crown hospitals," came into being slowly over the next half-century.

In 1818 the state levied a tax on every citizen over the entire country to finance a single class of hospitals to care for soldiers returning from the Napoleonic Wars (the last war the Swedes have fought). Many of them returned from their stay on the European continent with venereal disease, and the state assumed responsibility for their care. In addition, the state, with the cooperation of the Collegium Medicum, established a salaried health officer corps to serve not only the outlying areas but the cities as well. The responsibilities of these health officers went far beyond the treatment of venereal disease to the care of other communicable diseases as well, and they formed the basis for the current system of salaried district physicians.

Because Sweden was predominantly an agricultural country until well into the nineteenth century, social problems were usually worked out within the family, the village or the guild. A large number of guilds administered sickness insurance benefit programs; these in turn led to voluntary benevolent societies which began to flourish in the 1870s. Furthermore, the Local Government Reform of 1862 took the remaining burden of poor relief away from the church and made it the responsibility of the newly formed counties and municipalities, which were given taxing power. Medical care, already quite separate from poor relief because medical care was largely financed by the state and by insurance benefits, was definitively dissociated from it (unlike the situation in Britain and the United States), and local government was given the responsibility for the financing, maintenance and operation of general hospitals for all classes of people.

Between 1870 and 1930 Sweden underwent a period of rapid industrialization that radically changed the structure of the society and of its social-welfare system. During this period the proportion of workers employed in the agricultural sector dropped from 72 percent to 32 percent of all employed workers, and the proportion employed in industry rose from 15 percent to 36 percent. From 1850 to 1920 the emigration of over a million Swedes, mainly to the United States, was a reflection of the grinding rural poverty and urban unemployment that characterized much of Swedish life.

As industrialization increased, and as the family became less able to provide for its members in times of economic hardship or illness, a variety of social measures was enacted. The first occupational safety law was passed in 1889; in 1901 Parliament enacted a workmen's compensation law covering industrial accidents; and in 1918 a law was passed limiting the working day to eight hours. The first child-welfare legislation was enacted in 1902, and the Basic Pension Act was passed in 1913. But it was not until the depression of the 1930s that the national government became as deeply involved as it now is in all aspects of social welfare. Simultaneously there was rapid expansion of the medical-care system: Specialized county hospitals and less specialized local hospitals were built, and a system of district nurses was developed to supplement the already existing but limited system of district physicians.

In 1931 the government began to provide grants-in-aid to the voluntary sickness-benefit societies and a local voluntary health-insurance program was established. By 1954 almost 70 percent of the population was covered by sickness funds, and in 1955 all health-insurance funds were merged and a compulsory insurance system was founded under government control, guaranteeing income in case of illness. The Swedish health-insurance program thus developed on the basis of nonprofit sickness funds which were established in all parts of Sweden and were audited by government agencies. Later government subsidies provided additional funds, and when a large percentage of the population was covered, these programs were nationalized.

The county councils, which already had responsibility for general hospital care, were in 1951 given responsibility for the care of the chronically ill, who had previously received aid through the poor-relief system. In 1963 the county councils took over the system of district medical officers, and in 1967 the councils assumed responsibility for mental-health care. The counties thereby gained authority over most of Swedish medical care.

Organization of Sweden's Medical-Care System

Sweden's medical-care services are organized through a mixture of direct public ownership and provision of services, and reimbursement of costs through an employer-employee state-supported insurance system. The owners of most medical facilities and the contractors for most medical services, the county councils, cover 75 percent of Sweden's total health-care costs; the funding for this comes from local taxation (55 percent), fees charged for services, and allocation from the national government.

Compulsory contributions by employed workers, by employers and by the national government finance the national health-insurance plan, which is responsible for only a small part of hospital expenditures, but is responsible for most ambulatory care and for compensation of loss of earnings during illness; money spent by the national health-insurance plan accounts for some 10 percent of total health-care costs.

The national government, apart from its contributions to other levels of government, directly provides 14 percent of the costs—largely for specialized teaching hospitals and other central functions. Patients themselves pay out-of-pocket at the time of service only 1 percent of the total costs, in contrast to the United States where 33 percent of personal medical-care costs are paid directly by the patient.

Overall in 1970 the national government, the local government and the employer each paid about 30 percent of the costs of health service, and patient payments for health care, both through insurance and through out-of-pocket payments at the time of service, accounted for about 10 percent of the costs.

During the 1950s and 1960s the cost of medical care in Sweden rose rapidly. From 1950 to 1970 health-care expenditures in kronor, uncorrected for inflation, increased over tenfold. More significantly, in 1950 health-care costs in Sweden amounted to 3.2 percent of the GNP; by 1970 it had risen to 7 percent of the GNP, more than double its 1950 share. During that same period, in contrast, health-care costs in the United States rose from 4.6 percent of the GNP to 7.5 percent, and in Great Britain from 4.1 percent to only 4.9 percent, both considerably less than double the 1950 rate. This rise in Sweden, more rapid than in either of the other two countries, was due to exploding technical innovation in the health sector; the allocation of increased resources to specialist, hospital-based care; and to an increased demand for services, brought about by the rising standard of living and the changing pattern of morbidity.

Another factor in the high cost of Swedish medical care is the relatively high percentage of older people. Approximately 10 percent of the Swedish population is over 70, but this segment of the population uses about half of the hospital bed-days, including long-term-care beds. Persons over 80 comprise only 2.5 percent of the population but require 25 percent of all hospital care. And Sweden's aged population is increasing; it is estimated that by 1979 there will be an additional 100,000 people over 70, and that by 1985 one-eighth of the population will be over 70.

It has been established that people over 70 require not only 50 percent of the hospital care but also 25 percent of all other acute care, 30 percent of the psychiatric care and 75 percent of the available long-term care. Therefore, as the number of elderly grows, utilization and costs will also increase and the Swedish health-care system will be faced with even greater demands. At the same time there is expected to be a relative decrease in the size of the working population, which pays the costs.

During the late 1960s taxpayers began to express mounting unrest at the ever-increasing local taxes, and both local and national politicians and planners began to redefine health priorities. The Swedish response to exploding costs was planning, coordination and regionalization based on a voluntary approach: All sectors were invited to find a consensus and to act on it. During the late 1950s and early 1960s the formation of a Royal Commission on Regionalization was one of the first steps in encouraging the regionalization of hospital services. But according to some analysts, the voluntary approach simply led to the strengthening of the existing power structure and to protection of the status quo.

Since the early 1970s the planning machinery at the national level has been strengthened and major emphasis has been placed on control and regulation in the planning process. An effort is being made to give priority to ambulatory care over hospital care and, in part because of the relatively high prevalence of chronic disease, to the integration of hospital and ambulatory care with social services. There is evidence, however, that neither of these approaches has proven as successful as had been hoped.

Despite a 75 percent increase in the number of doctors from 1950 to 1965, Sweden still had fewer doctors per capita than other comparably wealthy countries. In 1970, 10,500 physicians were working in Sweden—a ratio of one physician for every 800 inhabitants. Through increased class size in Sweden's six medical schools, there was one doctor for each 600 people by 1975, about the same ratio as in the United States, and the current plan is to increase the number of doctors to 20,500, about one for every 450 people, by 1980. There are attempts to insure that a significant number of these physicians will work in primary care, and one method of insuring this lies in the power of the National Board of Health and Welfare to determine the number of training positions for each speciality as well as for general practice.

Overall, approximately 225,000 people—5.8 percent of the total labor force—were employed in health care in Sweden in 1973. This is a larger percentage than in the United States—5.1 percent in the same year. The difference lies mainly in the number of nonphysician health workers. In Sweden there were 15 other health workers for every physician; in the United States there were 12.

In 1972, 18 percent of the physicians, 29 percent of the dentists and 98 percent of the nurses and nurses' aides were women. The mean salaries for health workers in 1973 were: nonspecialist physicians—$25,200; specialist physicians—$30,600; district physicians—$31,600; dentists—$17,604; head nurses—$10,233; assistant nurses—$9,200; and nurses' aides—$7,431. These differences, already less than in the United States, are further reduced by a steeply progressive income tax.

The Swedish Parliament *(Riksdag),* a single-chamber parliament made up of 349 members who are elected every three years, has power over legislation, over the budget, and supervision of administration, but in practice it accepts the budget proposals and the administrative decisions of the executive branch. The real political power in Sweden lies with the prime minister and with his cabinet. Two sets of governmental bodies work under the prime minister: the ministries, which frame policy, and the national boards, which execute policy.

The Ministry of Health and Social Affairs, for example, prepares legislation in relation to health care, medical care and social services and prepares the government's health budget. The National Board of Health and Welfare cooperates in the planning at the national level and bears ultimate responsibility for supervision of Sweden's health care and medical care. This supervisory authority extends to both public and private facilities and regulates the work of physicians, nurses, midwives and other health workers.

The governmental level below the national level is the county *(län)*, with the county council *(landsting)* as the governing body. Twenty-three county councils and three municipal councils (Malmö, Göteborg and Gotland) are responsible for health services and hospital care and for education and social services. The level below the county is that of the 274 districts of local communities ("primary municipalities"), whose governing bodies are the municipal councils. The local district health centers, to which nursing homes and rehabilitation facilities are being attached more and more frequently, are, however, controlled at the county level. On the other hand, public health and social welfare are the responsibility of the "primary municipality"; cooperation between these two levels occurs at the local district health center.

Sweden has made significant efforts in the area of preventive health work. Environmental aspects of health are handled by a Public Health Board in each of Sweden's primary municipalities. This board is responsible for protection of the environment in such areas as food, sanitation, housing, air, water and noise. Some boards also take responsibility for health education, although this appears to remain a less developed area. Health education, which is provided in many settings such as schools, in the media and at hospitals, is aimed primarily at the public's eating, smoking, drinking and exercise habits.

Other preventive measures include the promotion of occupational health which is carried out through agreements between the labor unions and the employers' organization. Places of work with a large number of employees have access to nurses, physicians and safety engineers paid by the industry, and employees have significant input in assuring the safety of working conditions in the workplace.

Even in the provision of ambulatory care, Sweden's health-care system is heavily hospital-oriented. Sweden has a relatively low average (mean) number of physician visits per person per year—roughly three per person per year, which is a bit more than half the United States or the British rate. The Swedes somewhat make up for the relative paucity of physician visits by making many more visits directly to nurses than is the pattern in either the United States or Britain. Approximately 50 percent of doctor visits are to hospital outpatient departments where many of the physicians are specialists. Of the remainder, about half (25 percent of all physician visits) are to district physicians, and half (25 percent) to private practitioners.

Maternal and child health care is provided totally free of charge, almost entirely by the public sector. Maternity care is offered to all Swedish women, and since over 99 percent of all deliveries take place in the hospital, prenatal care is offered by both doctors and midwives in the hospital as well. Every newborn baby is visited at its home by the district nurse within a few days of birth; the provisions for care of the baby are discussed with the parents and any problems are dealt with. Care for children, including periodic checkups, immunizations, functional tests, and counseling, is provided by pediatric nurses, and when necessary by pediatricians, working in district child-care centers. It is estimated that 99.9 percent of newborn Swedish children are covered by these services, and this is believed to be one of the primary factors in Sweden's extremely low infant and maternal mortality rates. Further medical services to children are provided upon entering school and periodically throughout the school years.

Approximately 2000 district nurses work throughout Sweden, concentrating increasingly on care for the chronically sick, often older patient. Approximately 1000 district medical officers, usually general practitioners, work on salary outside of the hospitals under the administration of the county council. Their responsibilities are in many ways similar to those of British general practitioners—to provide primary medical care and preventive care to patients—but the population covered is a geographically defined district rather than a capitation panel. District physicians often work in solo practice, particularly in the sparsely populated northern areas, although the current trend is toward establishing larger districts where possible, with two or more physicians working in a center. A nurse or a nurse's aide usually works with the doctor, but district nurses also work independently, and problems of isolation—from each other and from other parts of the medical-care system—exist for both the district medical officers and the district nurses. The nursing district usually includes about half the population in a health district.

The financing for ambulatory care in Sweden is neither through a capitation system nor through a salaried system as it is in Great Britain (for primary care and for consultant care, respectively), but rather, as for most ambulatory care in the United States, on a payment-per-visit basis. Prior to January 1, 1970, if patients were seen on an ambulatory basis by a physician, even one employed by the county council, they had to pay the full cost of the fee and were then reimbursed 75 percent of what they paid. The patient, therefore, had to lay out the money, document the expenditures for reimbursement, and ended up paying at least 25 percent out of pocket. Reimbursement for laboratory tests and X rays was handled in the same way.

The 1970 reform attempted to simplify the administration of payment for ambulatory care by eliminating all economic transactions between patients and those doctors employed by the councils. For each ambulatory visit to a district health center or to a hospital, patients were required to pay seven Swedish kronor (about $1.75) and the national health insurance system would pay the rest. This amount has been gradually increased and is now 15 Swedish kronor ($3.75). At the same time, another reform was instituted which fixed salaries and working hours for the physicians who work for the county councils.

While there are very few private hospital beds and only slightly more private nursing home beds, roughly 10 percent (1500 out of 15,000) of the physicians in Sweden are in private practice. As indicated above, they handle about 25 percent of the ambulatory visits. When the patient sees a private doctor on an ambulatory basis, he now must pay 25 Swedish kronor ($6.25); the remainder of a fixed fee, negotiated by the Swedish Medical Association with the National Board of Health and Welfare, is covered by the compulsory health-insurance program.

It was not until 1973 that dental care was included under Sweden's health-insurance system, and eyeglasses are still not covered, although some counties have recently begun to provide glasses to children. The patient also pays part of the cost of medication, but a relatively small amount: 50 percent of the cost up to a maximum of 20 kronor (about $5). Herein lies an example of one of the tensions inherent in those parts of the system in which coinsurance plays a significant role. Since the maximum of 20 kronor applies to all prescriptions written for the patient on the same visit, patients not unexpectedly ask their physician to write as many prescriptions as possible at the same time, to write a single prescription for large quantities rather than sequential smaller prescriptions, and, occasionally, to write prescriptions actually meant for other members of the family, or other people, under the name of one patient. These abuses are not thought to be widespread, but illustrate potentials for problems.

Serious problems exist in the continuity of care between the ambulatory-care system and the hospital sector. As in England, primary-care physicians may not care for hospitalized patients except under special circumstances; physicians on the staffs of the hospitals take over the care once the patient is admitted. Despite efforts to provide the hospital physician with information about the patient and his problems, and to provide the primary-care physician with information about the hospitalization and its aftermath, confusion and discontinuity frequently exist.

The hospital sector has in recent years had the highest priority within the Swedish health system. Throughout the 1960s there was a high rate of hospital construction even though the overall occupancy rate declined from 85 percent in 1950 to 73 percent in 1968. Eighty percent of the operating expenses and 50 percent of the capital expenses go to the hospital sector from the county council. With 16 beds per 1000 population, Sweden has a very high ratio of beds to the size of its population; in comparison, the United States has 7 beds per 1000 population, and Great Britian 10 beds per 1000. Even if the comparison is limited to general hospital beds, Sweden's 7 per 1000 well exceeds the United States' and Britain's 5 per 1000.

It is of special interest, though, that the rate of admissions to Sweden's general hospitals (150 per 1000 people per year in 1970) is not very different from that in the United States (148 per 1000). The difference in use of general hospital beds comes in the length of stay: The average (mean) hospital stay in Sweden in 1970 was 12.7 days and in the United States 9.0 days. (In England and Wales, by contrast, admissions were only 102 per 1000 people per year and length of stay 10.8 days, a different pattern from either Sweden or the United States.) Overall, in 1970 Swedes had 1900 general hospital bed-days per 1000 population, Americans had 1300 per 1000, and Englishmen 1100 per 1000.

Why has Sweden made such a large investment in the hospital sector? A large part of the answer lies, of course, in its history. The age structure of Sweden's population may be another part of the explanation. Other factors include the political visibility of hospitals and related institutions, and the influence of the medical profession, particularly that segment which is based in academic institutions and in teaching hospitals. Some 70 to 75 percent of Sweden's physicians, and the vast majority of its nurses, work in hospitals—a large constituency for continued emphasis on hospital-based care.

All but a few of Sweden's 720 hospitals are run by county councils. The national government runs two hospitals—the Karolinska in Stockholm and the Akademiska sjukhuset in Uppsala, technologically unexcelled in the world—and there are three private hospitals.

Hospital care, including medical and surgical treatment, nursing, medicines and all auxiliary services, requires no direct out-of-pocket payment on the part of the patient. However, the hospitalized patient is charged 20 Swedish kronor ($5) per inpatient day and this amount is subtracted automatically from the daily insurance payments Swedes receive for loss of income when ill. Usually the individual is hospitalized in a local hospital which is administered by the county council. If the local hospital does not have the treatment needed, the county will pay the full cost of hospitalization in the central county hospital or the regional hospital.

Remaining Problems

While the Swedes are surely concerned with providing high-quality medical care to all of their people, while they are concerned with the problem of the high cost of medical care and the need for a greater emphasis on preventive medicine, on primary care and on regionalization of specialized and expensive resources, problems remain. One of these is the continuing problem of long waits for nonemergency ambulatory care; patients must often schedule appointments weeks or months in advance. There is a special problem in the accessibility to medical care in rural areas to which it is difficult to recruit district medical officers. The Swedes are attempting to deal with these problems by increasing the number of physicians and by encouraging them to practice in primary care rather than in specialities, but the problem of accessibility to care is far from solved.

Despite considerable attention to health care and a better record of devoting resources and social efforts to it than have most countries, many analysts feel that Sweden still spends a disproportionate amount of its resources on therapeutic medical care. Technological medical care, particularly for inpatients, has taken precedence over prevention and over ambulatory care, and it is difficult to reverse this trend in a society in which so much investment has been made in hospital facilities where so many health workers are employed.

A feature of the system with which the Swedes appear to be less concerned is the continued professional dominance of the physician. Teams consisting of different types of health workers do exist, both for inpatient care and ambulatory care, but the role of the physician as leader of the team in all its aspects seems to be relatively unquestioned except in mental health, where the role of the physician as leader has indeed been questioned. While movement toward worker management is markedly in evidence in many Swedish industries through the work-council system and is increasing in importance in many industries, it is not yet a strong force in the organization of medical-care institutions.

Furthermore, consumer participation in health care is not the issue in Sweden that it is in either the United States or in Great Britain. Where it does exist it consists largely of associations of people with certain diseases (*e.g.,* diabetes or kidney disease) acting as pressure groups for greater attention to research or care in their areas of interest. Of course, it is possible to claim that popular participation occurs through the county councils which provide and finance most of the health services. But while such participation may indeed take place, it is surely not as direct and intense a participation as is being attempted by community health councils in England and by some instances of consumer participation in health care in the United States, not to speak of the extremely different order of involvement of people in China.

A further issue is whether health services in Sweden are a factor for or against equity. Approximately 60 percent of the funds used for the payment of health services are collected by proportional taxation—55 percent collected by the county councils from personal income tax revenues and approximately 5 percent from employer-employee funds. Since proportional taxation—taxation in which the tax rate remains constant regardless of the level of income—usually places a greater burden on the poor who must pay the tax with income needed for basic expenses, it is said to be "regressive" in its effect on equitable distribution of income.

Of course, it must be remembered that taxation for health services is only a small part of total taxation in Sweden, and that the bulk of the tax pattern, and the service pattern outside medicine, is heavily redistributive. Furthermore, since there are relatively few barriers, geographic or financial, to the use of health services in Sweden, utilization seems relatively equitably distributed among all groups in society in relation to their needs.

Overall, health and medical care, along with Sweden's high standard of living, seem to be among the contributing factors to the extraordinarily good health of the Swedish people. Sweden has developed a medical system which is a strong and reasonably efficient and effective part of its health-promotion and human-service system. It contributes, though not as much as it could, to equity and community, and is one model for attempting to deal with some of these problems in a pluralistic, highly technological and highly professionalized society.

3

GREAT BRITAIN— Equitable Entitlement

Great Britain, a society whose economy is also mixed but significantly less affluent than Sweden's, has emphasized universal entitlement and preservation of the family doctor through a national health service.

The Setting

Great Britain is of special interest to us because it is a society whose basic economic structure, values, language and culture are close to our own, and yet a society that chooses to organize and pay for its medical-care services in a way quite different from ours. The British National Health Service, initiated in 1948, has protected—some would say "frozen"—a system of medical care based on the general practitioner, who still practices a personal style of primary care that has become extinct in most of the United States. This care, and almost all medical care for everyone who finds himself in Great Britain, from the longest-lived inhabitant to the newly arrived tourist, is paid for through tax funds with essentially no cost to the patient at the time of the service.

On the other hand, and this comes as a shock to most Americans—and Britons, too, for that matter—the United Kingdom (Great Britain and Northern Ireland) is now a relatively poor country with severe economic problems. Not only is its GNP per capita low among the industrialized countries of the world ($3800, compared to $7900 for Sweden and $7100 for the United States, in 1975), but the fraction of that GNP which it allots to health care is also low compared to that of other countries.

Patients, however, seem quite satisfied with their "National Health." The reasons are easy to discern: Britons for the most part have available to them accessible, responsive, humane, technically competent health care and medical care.

The features of the British National Health Service that are most relevant to our discussion include: (1) the elimination of financial barriers to access to all medical care, including primary care; (2) the organizational tactics which were felt to be necessary in order to gain the cooperation of both the general practitioners and the specialists when the service was introduced, and the changes that have been made since; (3) the continuing attempts to make the system and its impact more equitable; (4) the efforts to provide medical care in a community context and to enable community members to participate more fully in the health-care system; and (5) the preservation of a community-based primary-care physician who provides accessible, integrated and continuing care for the ambulatory patient, usually on a family basis.

Most of the description of health- and medical-care services in this chapter refers to the situation in England and Wales. Scotland (the other major component of Great Britain) is served by the National Health Service, but it is separately administered and differs, although usually in relatively small and subtle ways, from its southerly counterpart.

Preservation of the Family Doctor

A family in Liverpool or London, in Horton-in-Ribblesdale in Yorkshire or other hamlets in rural Britain, from the youngest member with a common cold to the eldest with a chronic, disabling disease, will, in all likelihood, receive its primary health care from a local general practitioner. The "GP" (a term often used disparagingly in the United States but usually descriptively or respectfully in Britain) generally knows the family and is familiar with the environment in which it lives.

The GP's office (or "surgery" as it is called, although little surgery is performed there) usually reflects the milieu in which it is situated and therefore varies markedly from area to area. There are those in Bloomsbury and Belgravia with bright brass nameplates on the outer door and elegant dark paneled rooms inside; others, in the poorer sections of the inner-London borough of Camden, for example, are in cold, dingy, meagerly furnished storefronts; and some, increasingly being built throughout Britain, are in modern, bustling, technologically well-equipped health centers. In recent years more and more GPs have installed appointment systems, which tend to lessen the patients' waiting time, but waiting rooms are still often crowded with people sitting patiently, waiting to be seen.

GPs provide primary medical care to those who are registered with them; they do not restrict their work to any special age or sex, disease or system. Individuals are free to register with any GP of their choosing, provided only that the GP is willing to accept them on his/her list. The GP provides first contact and long-term continuing care; it has been estimated that the GP is the only point of contact for 90 percent of the episodes of ill health for which physician help is sought in Britain. Patients suffering "minor" or chronic illnesses will most likely be treated solely by the GP; patients with "major" or complex illnesses are usually referred for consultation and possibly treatment to a specialist clinic at the hospital. Most contact with specialists is made through the GP, who also utilizes other medical and community resources for the care of the patient.

The GP is paid by the National Health Service through an annual capitation fee for each patient on his list; in 1975 the average (mean) list size was approximately 2300 patients. Since Britons have a relatively low mobility rate compared to that of the United States, and since British GPs see almost 75 percent of all patients on their lists at least once a year and at least one member from 90 percent of all families on their lists at least once each year, GPs get to know many of their patients rather well. Furthermore, while patients are free to leave their GP and register with another, fewer than 1 percent of patients change their physicians in any given year because of dissatisfaction.

General practitioners have considerable leeway in organizing their work: They may provide their own premises, hire their own staff and equip their own offices. They may work singly, in two-person partnerships or in larger groups; the strong trend in recent years, however, has been toward working in groups. The GP may or may not work directly with nonphysician personnel in the same premises, though the current trend, fostered by financial incentive, is to do so. And more and more GPs are practicing in health centers, where the local public health workers join them in the care of patients from a defined geographic district.

While GPs themselves often express considerable dissatisfaction with the system, the public, as poll after poll has shown, invariably expresses considerable satisfaction with it. In any case, it is the GP who is the cornerstone of the British healthcare system. A strong investment has been made in the maintenance of locally based, continuing, integrated, personal care—and it seems to work.

Historical Background

The development of the current British health system has been a gradual, evolutionary one. The creation of the National Health Service in 1948 was not the sharp, radical break with the past it has sometimes been pictured as in the United States; it was rather a logical outgrowth of the past organization of medical care when confronted with mid-twentieth-century British politics and with rapid advances in science and technology.

Indeed, the roots of the present British National Health Service, and its problems as well, extend back several hundred years into the historical development of the medical profession and the hospital. The differences in the status of consultants and general practitioners have been a cause of concern since the sixteenth century; current hospital staffing patterns evolved in voluntary teaching hospitals in the eighteenth and nineteenth centuries; the referral system by general practitioners to specialists was developed by the two groups of doctors in the late nineteenth century to eliminate competition between them for patients; and the divergence in resources between London and the provinces and between teaching and nonteaching hospitals is centuries old.

As early as the sixteenth century the importance of the professional association as the arbiter of medical standards in Britain was apparent. In 1518 the Royal College of Physicians of London was incorporated by Henry VIII to oversee the practice of medicine within a seven-mile radius of the city of London. While the reason given for the establishment of the Royal College was to protect the public from charlatans by licensing recognized physicians in order to distinguish them from unqualified practitioners, in fact the accredited physicians attended only the royal family, the aristocracy and the wealthy, and were themselves drawn from the upper strata of society. A monopoly over medical care was thereby established, with the College the exclusive domain of upper-class medical practitioners, a professional guild of and for the elite.

The role of the professional association was reinforced by the development of an apprenticeship system of training. Medical schools were founded by practicing doctors to enhance their reputations, their practices and their fees; and hospitals, which were small and few in number and played a relatively minor role in the total provision of medical care, nonetheless became valuable places for the teaching of apprentices and in some instances for research, as well as for lucrative practice.

Specialist practice was organized around specific diseases or specific organ systems rather than around the patient's overall care needs. Hospital staffing was as much or more influenced by the pattern of bedside teaching as by the need of the patients for care. A small, elite group of doctors was attached to each voluntary hospital, and a group of hospital beds was assigned to a specific doctor who was responsible for the treatment of the patients in them. The bed group became a semiautonomous unit, where patients with similar conditions were kept together on one ward under one doctor's aegis. Each physician or surgeon had his own retinue and used the patients for the teaching of medical students at the bedside.

During the 1800s, physicians felt themselves to be the "cream" of society and they and the surgeons looked upon the hospital as their property rather than the public's. Consequently in the nineteenth century, in marked contrast to the continental pattern, medical schools developed around these voluntary hospitals rather than around universities, and teaching and research served primarily to increase the prestige of the practicing doctor.

The people who were not treated by the increasingly hospital-based physicians and surgeons often went to a local drug dispenser or apothecary for their medical care. Apothecaries were originally general shopkeepers, but they assumed a separate identity when they broke away from the Mystery of Grocers in 1617. The apothecary's right to treat the sick was established during the plague of 1665 when physicians, along with their affluent patients, moved out of the city, leaving the rest of the citizenry to the care of the apothecaries. The House of Lords in the early eighteenth century, over the objections of the Royal College of Physicians of London, upheld the apothecaries' right to treat the sick, and the apothecaries gradually extended their medical activities from keeping chemists' shops, where they compounded physicians' prescriptions, to selling over-the-counter drugs, to treating and prescribing for patients in their homes.

The following notice, displayed in the window of an apothecary's shop in Manchester during the early 1800s, illustrates the diverse functions of the apothecary:

> Surgeon and Apothecary. Prescriptions and family medicines accurately compounded. Teeth extracted at one shilling each. Women attended in labour, two shillings and sixpence each. Patent medicines and perfumery. Best London pickles. Fish sauces. Bear's grease. Soda water. Ginger beer, Lemonade, Congreve's matches and Warren's blackening.

The position of "resident apothecary" was developed in the eighteenth-century voluntary hospital to help the physician to care for his patients, but for the most part the role of the apothecary was entirely outside the hospital. In 1815, three centuries after the first specialists' society was founded, the Society of Apothecaries was given power to examine and license apothecaries throughout England and Wales. Apothecaries became relatively well trained and informed medical practitioners, though they were nonetheless still educationally and socially inferior to the small elite of physicians. As the profession developed, the physicians and surgeons began to call themselves consultants, and apothecaries began to call themselves general practitioners.

By the mid–nineteenth century, when the Medical Act of 1858 established a single medical register for all medical practitioners with recognized diplomas or degrees and institutionalized the three separate categories of doctor (physician, surgeon and apothecary) the general practitioner was firmly established as the doctor of first and continuing contact for the rising middle classes. The British Medical Association, founded during this period as a successor to an older Provincial Medical and Surgical Association, was to become, in opposition to the London-based Royal Colleges, the champion of the general practitioner and his spokesman for higher recognition.

The power of consultant physicians and surgeons was vastly increased by the scientific study of disease during the first half of the nineteenth century. Specialty hospitals began to develop to facilitate this study and led to increases in the number of specialists. Toward the end of the nineteenth century specialty departments were established in general hospitals, and the growth of cities and towns fostered the formation of specialist practices, which could survive only in large populations. Consultant physicians and surgeons had access to beds in the voluntary hospitals; general practitioners, without such access, generally had lower incomes and an inferior status, at least within the profession.

The urbanization of the nineteenth century and the attendant rise of the middle class strengthened the position of the general practitioner because the specialist physicians at first ignored this market. They soon began to compete for the patronage of the newly prospering middle class, and the specialists' standing in the hospitals—the centers of medical technical innovation— gave them an edge on the GP. The competition, however, threatened to be disadvantageous to both groups of doctors, and by the end of the nineteenth century a referral system had evolved through informal professional agreement: Hospital-based doctors would act as consultants, while the general practitioner retained the primary relationship with the patient. As one observer has described this relationship, "The physician and surgeon retained the hospital, but the general practitioner retained the patient." The specialist physician, however, still retained the care for the very well-to-do in his private consulting rooms in Harley Street and in the equivalents in the provincial towns.

Intersecting with the evolution of the pattern of medical practice was the evolution of care for the poor. The first Elizabethan Poor Law, in 1601, made the local parish responsible for the relief of the destitute using tax levy funds, and workhouses were built to house the old, the sick, widows and orphans. Much of the care of the poor remained, however, in the hands of the aristocracy as a matter of *noblesse oblige* toward those living on their estates or working in their service.

It also became customary for the successful industrialist or trader to bequeath money to found a hospital or dispensary.

Thus, most hospitals were built not under the aegis of government—as in Sweden, where there was therefore some attempt at equitable distribution—but on the private initiative of, and therefore at locations chosen by, the upper classes. Ultimately the boards of governors of these hospitals were drawn from among those who could support the hospital financially and the boards became socially prestigious. One of the privileges of membership was the receipt of tickets which could be given at the members' discretion to poor people, entitling them to admission to the hospital for care; these were usually given to those regarded as the "deserving poor."

With the Poor Law reform of 1834—one of a long series—the responsibilities of the parishes were grouped into larger units under Poor Law boards, which were the forerunners of the present Ministry of Health. As the cities grew (by 1850 one-half of the population of England lived in the cities, the first nation on earth to reach this point), these boards hired workhouse medical officers and district medical officers for the care of sick paupers.

Thus by the turn of the century there was a three-class structure of medical care in Britain: The paupers were cared for in the municipal hospitals; the poor in voluntary hospitals; and the well-off in private hospitals or, more likely, at home with the constant attendance of servants.

The Public Health Act of 1848 which established a central organizing body, the General Board of Health, was the first direct acknowledgment of the state's responsibility for control of environmental hazards to health. But it was not until the Public Health Act of 1875 that effective public health institutions were firmly established in Britain. During the last quarter of the nineteenth century and the beginning of the twentieth century, most of the new medical officers of health were part-time general practitioners. They were responsible for a wide variety of duties such as the certification of births and deaths; the reporting of infectious disease; vaccinations; and the care of children.

When workmen's compensation legislation was instituted, GPs were called in to legitimate claims for injuries. Many were also under contract to trade unions and "friendly societies" to provide medical care to the members and to certify their claims to the cash benefits these organizations were providing. Many GPs found that these tasks brought them into conflict with their professional ethics, and this conflict finally persuaded them to support the move for a state-based health-insurance plan. Many also felt that the British Medical Association no longer represented their interests. They therefore formed a trade union—the Medical Practitioners Union—part of whose policy it was to support establishment of state-run medical services. Thus the health and social problems that were the legacy of the world's first Industrial Revolution were part of the impetus for governmental health insurance.

Direct state involvement in the financing of medical services began with the Health Insurance Act of 1911. This act focused solely on general practitioner services and thereby further emphasized the division between the general practitioner and the consultant. It financed the primary medical care of most employed manual workers who were compulsorily covered. An upper level was set for income as a qualification for eligibility, and the payment mechanism chosen for the GP was capitation—the payment of a fixed annual fee for each patient on the GP's list, no matter how frequently or how seldom the patient consulted the doctor. The effect of the act was to consolidate and strengthen the position of the general practitioner, to increase their numbers and to bolster the referral system.

Other important pre–World War I legislation included the development of a school health service—including free or subsidized school meals for poor children—and legislation which permitted, and then mandated, local authorities to establish maternity and child-health, midwifery and community nursing services. Thus, by World War I the basic pattern of current health services and of medical practice in Britain had been established.

In 1920 a consultative council to the Ministry of Health of England and Wales, under the chairmanship of Lord Dawson of Penn, issued an "Interim Report on the Future of Medical and Allied Services." In its recommendations the report was far ahead of its time, calling for the establishment of "primary health centers" which, at one site, would provide a combination of primary medical care by general practitioners and health care by health workers responsible for community-based preventive services. The concept, however, was interpreted by GPs as requiring the integration of the GP's work with the work of the local health authority—with a consequent diminution of the GP's autonomous role—and it was strongly resisted.

During the 1920s and 1930s, hospitals increasingly became centers for "scientific medicine" and the number of specialists grew rapidly. Because of the number of personnel and the amount of complex equipment needed in a specialist environment, hospital costs also rose rapidly. In 1929–30 the Poor Law infirmaries were taken over by local authorities. In theory they were general hospitals, but in fact most of them housed the aged and the chronically ill. There was little or no coordination between them and the voluntary hospitals, and little or no regional planning.

On the other hand, by 1938, 40 percent of the total population of England and Wales was covered for ambulatory-care services and cash sickness benefits by the Health Insurance Act of 1911, and 90 percent of all general practitioners were participating in the system. General practitioners, whose income and status had been raised by national health insurance, were, on the whole, favorable to the system, and the British Medical Association and other medical organizations recognized the need for its extension to other workers and their dependents.

Each year the technical gap—as well as the prestige and income gap—between the consultant physician or surgeon and the GP grew wider. Yet the great majority of practicing doctors in England and Wales continued to be general practitioners, often having their surgeries or offices in the front room of their own homes. In 1939, for example, there was one full-time consultant to every six or seven British general practitioners, but more than one-third of those specialists practiced in London.

As World War II neared, there was a growing need to deal with some of the outstanding issues in the provision of medical care: (1) Insurance coverage was inadequate, both in the number of people uncovered and in the limited scope of benefits; (2) hospital development and the provision of specialist services were chaotic; (3) general practice was provided in inefficient and often technically inadequate ways; and (4) there was conflict between the roles of the general practitioner and the consultant.

The National Health Service

World War II gave great impetus to the establishment of a national health service. At the outbreak of the war in 1939 an emergency medical service was formed which became involved in three crucial areas: regional planning, the focusing of particular services in specialist centers, and the assigning of medical staff to teaching and municipal hospitals. It had significant impact on the attitude of the medical profession toward the reorganization of hospital facilities and ultimately on the long-term organization of medical care.

Another impetus toward the establishment of a national health service was the 1942 Beveridge Report, which made far-reaching recommendations for services from "the cradle to the grave." The report formed the basis of the postwar system of social-welfare reforms, and held as a central assumption that a comprehensive system of health care and medical care was essential to any plan for improving living standards. The rationale was both an ideological commitment to equity and the expectation that the expenditure on improved medical care would be self-liquidating because it would produce a healthier nation. (This expectation, it should be noted, has largely proved false in every country because, among other factors, it exaggerates the effect of medical care on health, neglects the effects of an aging population and higher prevalence of chronic illness, and assumes incorrectly that demand for care is equivalent to need for care.)

The enactment of legislation establishing a national health service was assured by the 1945 election of a Labor government and the subsequent naming of Aneurin Bevan as minister of health. During the planning with the government to determine the shape of the new health service, the consultants were more receptive than the general practitioners since they felt they had more power and more room to maneuver. The general practitioners had several qualms, including the fear that they would be placed on a basic salary and therefore would be "reduced" to the status of civil servants. The consultants were induced to accept the new system by extraordinary fringe benefits and perquisites attached to their salaried status—including the possibility of working part-time on salary and part-time for private fees. Although Bevan believed at the time that these concessions were necessary, he is quoted as having claimed that he "stuffed the mouths of the consultants with gold."

The general practitioners were brought into the National Health Service by permitting them to remain "independent contractors" under a capitation system rather than join it as salaried employees. Another price paid for securing the cooperation of various interests, including those of the local authorities, was that "preexisting administrative and professional divisions between the historical branches of practice were to be widened, not abolished." Patients in the community were to be under the care of general practitioners, and all hospital patients were to be under the care of the specialists. It was originally planned that general practitioners would increasingly practice in health centers to reduce their isolation and integrate their work with preventive service, but little incentive toward the development of health centers was provided. Local government control over community health services was maintained. In short, Bevan's goal of an integrated health service, as opposed to a disease-treatment service, was not realized.

With regard to hospitals, both the small voluntary hospitals and the municipal hospitals were to be nationalized and operated by 14 regional hospital boards. The university teaching hospitals would be administered by boards of governors who retained control of their endowment funds and had direct access to the Ministry of Health. Consultants and specialists were to be employed by the regional hospital board, or by the boards of governors in the case of the teaching hospitals, and private practice was to be permitted for part-time consultants.

The National Health Service Act of 1948 therefore created a tripartite organizational structure around traditional patterns of care: a hospital service, with specialists salaried in all but name; general medical, ophthalmic and dental care, on a contractual basis; and local preventive and supportive services provided by the health departments of local government. These three arms were coordinated only at the national level, that of the Ministry of Health. Furthermore, many of the problems that had existed prior to the establishment of the National Health Service still remained, particularly the disparity in rewards between specialists and general practitioners and the disparity in services between teaching and nonteaching hospitals.

On the "appointed day," July 5, 1948, the British National Health Service Act was implemented. It guaranteed health care for all without charge at the time of care irrespective of income level. Eleven thousand specialists and other doctors working in hospitals and 18,000 general practitioners entered the National Health Service on that day, against the advice of the British Medical Association. The medical profession as a whole, however, had emerged as a strong force from the negotiations surrounding the Act; at each level of administration there was substantial medical representation. According to one observer at the time, "As a profession . . . we are in a more powerful position than ever before."

Freedom of choice was upheld for the doctors: They could participate in the service, were free to take private patients as well, and no interference was permitted in their "clinical judgment." Freedom of choice was also largely upheld for the patients: They could use the service or go to doctors outside the service, but in either case they still paid for the service through their taxes. They could choose their GP, but except in emergencies the choice of and referral to specialists was to be made by the GP. Despite the increased formal restrictions (which really made relatively little difference in practice from previous patterns of care), the idea of medical care free to everyone at the time of service was a popular one and, all in all, the National Health Service was absorbed quickly into British life.

The National Health Service brought a clear division between the administration and financing of hospital and specialist services and that of general-practice services, and most immediate post-1948 developments favored the specialist rather than the general practitioner. Society had become specialty-conscious, not only in medical care but in all fields, and the number of specialists and of junior hospital staff in training to become specialists increased steadily. The main advances after World War II in medical science were made in teaching hospitals and not in general practice, and hospital care became more technological and more expensive year by year.

The status of consultants under the National Health Service rose dramatically from their already high status prior to the implementation of the Act. Their fringe benefits—such as vacations, pensions, sick leave, study leave and, most important, the opportunity to earn distinction awards—significantly increased their income. They simultaneously exerted great influence and retained flexibility; many worked just short of full-time for the service and were therefore free to earn as much as they could in lucrative private practice on their own time; they could even use Health Service facilities in the hospitalization of their private patients. From 1948 until the reorganization of the National Health Service in 1974, the consultants generally expressed more satisfaction in the National Health Service than did the general practitioners.

Indeed, the effect of the National Health Service on the general practitioner was initially quite different. General practitioners were virtually excluded from practice in the larger hospitals (although some small "cottage" hospitals were open to them). Furthermore, the concept of health centers, which had been a central theme during the negotiations for the National Health Service, had largely disappeared after its implementation. The prestige of a newly established Royal College of General Practitioners in 1952 helped to increase the satisfaction and prestige of those GPs who became members, but most of the GPs felt isolated, excluded from the high technology (where the "action" was), underrespected and underpaid relative to the consultants. After an initial decline in their numbers, they succeeded in the mid-1960s in promoting reforms which, through financial and organizational changes, increased their incomes, encouraged the hiring of staff such as nurses to the practice, and encouraged them to practice in groups. At the same time local authorities were allowed to build health centers in which GPs could work together with district nurses, social workers and other staff supplied by the local health authority.

Despite its problems, the creation of the National Health Service, in the words of one observer, "represented a radical change in the relationship between the individual citizen and the State, and it established a firm government commitment to developing and improving the country's system of health care." The major achievements of the Act were (1) to provide medical care free of charge on the basis that need, rather than ability to pay, ought to govern access to care, and (2) to allow for at least the possibility of rationalizing the provision of resources at national and local levels.

Community-based primary care and preventive services are an important part of the system. In addition to the general practitioner, a wide variety of health workers provides care in the community. Much of the work is done by medical and nursing staff who see patients at preventive clinics on a sessional basis. A "domiciliary" service is provided by home nurses to patients who need nursing care. Health visitors, who are nurses with additional specialized training in social aspects of health education, also play a significant role in the provision of primary and preventive care. They are statutorily required to visit every mother after the birth of a baby and continue to observe the baby's development until it is five years of age; they also visit families to give advice on a wide variety of health matters and serve as a vital link between individuals and the health and social-service departments.

Medical diagnosis and treatment are in the hands of the GP, most of whose work is concerned with "common and minor illnesses." According to a study done in 1970–71, 62 percent of the patient visits to a GP are for "minor illnesses" with little or no risk of loss of life or of permanent disability; 13 percent involve "major illnesses" and these patients are usually referred for treatment to a specialist at the hospital; and 25 percent are for "chronic conditions." Although access to the GP is usually fairly easy, one study showed that 75 percent of symptoms are treated by the patients themselves without going to see any doctor. The average patient consults the GP four times a year; those who consult him more frequently tend to be the old, the young, people who live alone, and members of particular "at risk" occupational groups such as miners.

Adding in the visits to specialists (roughly two per person per year), it is clear that the fact that care is free at the time of use has not, as many had predicted, vastly escalated the demand for care. Quite the contrary, it appears that the rate of ambulatory physician visits in Britain (4.9 per person per year in 1972), where an exceedingly small proportion involve direct payment, is very close to the rate in the United States (5.0 per person per year in 1973, including telephone), where many of the visits involve direct payment by the patient. Furthermore, there is evidence that the working class in Britain makes substantially more use of the system than does the middle class—a consequence of the system's emphasis on equity—even though some argue that middle-class people still seem able to manipulate the system more to meet their needs than do those who are poorer.

The current trend is for the general practitioner to work more closely with other GPs and with nonphysician personnel.

Approximately 45 percent of all general practitioners today work in groups of three or more doctors. In addition, most general practitioners employ a secretary or a receptionist; and health visitors, midwives, home nurses and social workers who are paid by the local authority are also more and more frequently attached to practices. In groups, consultation with other GPs is readily available, and a team approach to medical care is facilitated by having representatives of several different health disciplines under the same roof.

Health centers which house a group of physicians, usually five or six, plus other health workers, are now increasing rapidly in number. Although the original National Health Service Act provided for health centers, only 28 were built in England from 1948 to 1967. Because of new finances made available to local authorities, 250 new health centers were opened between 1967 and 1971, and by 1975 there were almost 600. In the health center the model of coordination of preventive and treatment services, originally proposed by Lord Dawson in 1920, is finally being realized.

The income gap between GPs and consultants has narrowed since 1967 and a GP's lifetime earnings can now exceed those of a full-time NHS consultant specialist. In addition to the basic capitation payment for each person on his list, the contract agreed upon in 1967 gave the GP a higher capitation rate per patient if he has between 2500 and 3500 patients, and extra remuneration for each person over 65, for taking night calls, for care of persons who stay only temporarily in the GP's area, for maternity care, for family planning services, and for certain preventive measures. GPs also receive partial reimbursement for salaries of receptionists/secretaries and nurses and for rent spent on the premises. Extra payments are also made for seniority, postgraduate education, approved vocational training, for working in groups of three or more physicians from common premises, and for working in areas that are underdoctored. In short, the incentives are intended to strengthen preventive services for everyone, to expand medical services for those least well served in the past, and to facilitate access to care.

The NHS integrated the hospitals and reduced, even if it did not eliminate, the distinctions between the old voluntary and the old municipal hospitals. Beds were—and in many instances still are—likely to be arranged in large wards according to specialties. Patients are admitted to the hospital by consultants (or by junior staff working under their supervision) on referral from the general practitioners, usually from a waiting list, or directly from the hospital accident and emergency departments. In the hospital the patient becomes the responsibility of a "firm" which is made up of a consultant and a number of junior doctors, the latter comparable in many ways to "residents" (house staff) in the United States.

After discharge the patient, in principle, again becomes the responsibility of his GP, although in practice there is often considerable overlap and at times confusion about responsibility for specific aspects of continuing specialty care. Lack of communication between GP and consultant is seen as a continuing problem.

Thus, despite the great advance in equity and the preservation of a viable system of primary care, serious problems continued to exist. The uneven distribution of services prior to 1948, although markedly lessened, was not eradicated by the creation of the National Health Service; the demand for National Health Service care rose rapidly and resources were often insufficient to meet the need; the predominance of hospital service pushed general practice and preventive medicine into the background; there was little opportunity for community participation in the system, nor for accountability to the community; and the tripartite division of the service—operated by three sets of bodies having relatively little connection with one another at the local level—led to waste and frustration.

The National Health Service Reorganization of 1974

As early as 1962 there began to be serious discussion about the need for reorganization of the National Health Service in order to achieve a more equitable and rational deployment of resources. After several studies and formal reports, the National Health Service Reorganization Act was passed by Parliament, and given Royal Assent on July 5, 1973, exactly 25 years after the original "appointed day."

The objectives of the reorganization included unification of the three branches of the National Health Service and, by a redrawing of NHS administrative boundaries to match those of local authorities, the provision of mechanisms for closer collaboration between the local authorities, who provide much of the social and preventive services, and the medical professionals. In addition, since planning was to be done by appointed rather than elected authorities and much of it was centralized, there was an attempt to provide a vehicle for consumer participation through newly established community health councils.

At the head of the reorganized structure is the secretary of state for social services who is ultimately responsible to Parliament for the provision of health services. The secretary is assisted by junior ministers and civil servants at the Department of Health and Social Security, primarily a planning and administrative body which assists the secretary of state in deciding on national health objectives and priorities as well as matters concerned with National Health Service finance, personnel, and regional development.

Fourteen regional health authorities (RHAs), covering regions which may exceed three million people, comprise the next level of administrative authority. Their primary task is to arrange the distribution of the region's health services in accordance with nationally and regionally determined policies. The regional medical officer, for example, is responsible for planning the distribution of medical manpower in the region and for insuring that medical education and research facilities are developed sufficiently to meet the needs of the region. The RHAs have taken over the functions of the old regional hospital boards—the planning of hospital and consultant services, the appointment of hospital staff, and the distribution of clinical work among the hospitals within the region.

Detailed planning and organizing of day-to-day work is the responsibility of 90 area health authorities, an average of 6 per region. The AHAs are intended to be the embodiment of an integrated health service. The areas of responsibility, usually identical in boundaries with those of the metropolitan "districts" and the nonmetropolitan counties, range from under 250,000 people in some city areas to over one million in some rural counties.

The area health authorities have the dual responsibility of planning and of providing comprehensive health services, including hospital, community and domiciliary care, for the people of their area. Furthermore, the AHAs are delegated responsibility to study the health needs of the area, to determine where services fall below required standards, to collaborate with local authorities in providing social services, to be concerned with health education, and to set up the Family Practitioner Committee which deals with the work of general practitioners, dentists, pharmacists and opticians. While family practitioners are still independent contractors, administered separately from hospitals and community services, the family practitioner services administrator for an area is accountable to the area administrator. This relationship is an attempt to bring this aspect of the service closer to the rest of the National Health Service than was possible when the only accountability to other elements of the service was at the national level.

Districts, which range in population from 85,000 to 500,000, about three per area, are the next level of organization, the level at which community health services are provided. The services, which are run by district management teams, include clinics for expectant and nursing mothers, district general hospitals, child health and school health examinations, family planning, vaccinations and immunizations.

A further outgrowth of the 1974 reorganization was the creation at the district level of community health councils (CHCs) which were developed in order to provide local consumer participation in a system that was fundamentally built upon centralized professional planning. The CHCs provide for representation of users' views, but administrative responsibility is left in the hands of the appointed health authorities. Half of the CHC members are appointed directly by the local authorities, and one-third are nominated by voluntary organizations. The remaining one-sixth are chosen by the regional health authorities from people who are supposed to have particular knowledge of health issues. The issues considered to be within the purview of the CHCs include:

> the effectiveness of services being provided; the planning of services; collaboration between the health services and local authorities; assessing the extent to which district health facilities conform with the published Departmental policies; the share of available resources devoted to the care of patients unable to protect their own interests . . . ; facilities for patients; waiting periods; quality of catering; and monitoring the volume and type of complaints received about a service or institution.

As one observer has noted, "The list would require the ideal CHC member to spend considerable time mastering the data needed to carry out his or her task of assessing standards, investigating conditions and getting involved in the planning process." And all this without any direct administrative authority or responsibility.

Evaluation of the work of the CHCs is still premature. Many CHC reports complain bitterly of public ignorance of their existence, while other groups have demonstrated that the general public will respond if the CHC provides a specific service. Some observers feel that the CHCs are essentially powerless; others point out that the National Health Service is a virtual monopoly in which the delivery of services is the responsibility of professionals who are accountable only to other professionals, and that the CHCs have at least "widened the political arena within which discussions about the allocation and use of NHS resources take place."

The vast majority of the financing for the National Health Service—over 80 percent—comes out of "progressive" (increasing-rate-with-increasing-income) general taxation. Less than 10 percent comes through "regressive" (flat-rate-regardless-of-income) social security payments. Direct payments for services received, such as for some dental services and a small fixed charge for each prescription, contribute less than 5 percent. The preponderance of tax levy funds is both a strength and a weakness of the system. It provides a much more equitable way of paying for health services than flat-rate social security payments or other models (including the one used in Sweden); but it also means that health care and medical care have to compete with other services, such as education, for the allocation of tax monies. Many feel that in Britain health care and medical care have come out second best, or considerably lower, in the political struggle for priorities.

Public satisfaction with the system is seen not only in the public opinion polls, but in the relatively small reliance on the private sector in medicine by those who could pay for it. Private health-insurance plans, and direct payment to private doctors, indeed exist. In fact there has been some increase in membership in private insurance plans in the last few years. But these are largely the result of industry offering this as a tax shelter and perquisite to groups of managerial employees and not necessarily reflective of dissatisfaction with the NHS. Private practice is used largely for "convenience"—extra privacy or extra privileges, such as jumping the waiting list for "minor" medicine and surgery. When someone in Britain is seriously ill, it is almost invariably the National Health Service that is used. Overall, only about 2 percent of medical expenditures in Britain are in private medicine.

Medical education in Britain, as in the United States, is based largely on academic rather than practice models. In recent years there have been 10 to 20 applicants for each of the 3500 medical-school places, and the successful applicants are chosen largely on the basis of their Advanced Level examination scores in the premedical sciences—physics, chemistry and biology.

The first two or three years of undergraduate medical education, devoted to preclinical sciences, are usually taught in a university medical school by nonclinicians, with little or no contact with patients. Then follows three years of clinical education in university teaching hospitals. After these five or six years the student is graduated as an M.B., Ch.B. (Bachelor of Medicine, Bachelor of Surgery). The M.D. degree in Britain is an advanced research degree based on the submission of a thesis; very few doctors in Britain have obtained the degree. The undergraduate education of the student is estimated to cost $2000 to $4000 per year, but payment is highly subsidized and the maximum direct payment by the student is about $1200 per year.

After passing qualifying examinations, the student is provisionally registered with the General Medical Council and works for a year as a junior member of the hospital staff, six months on a medical unit and six months on a surgical unit. At the end of this period he is fully registered with the General Medical Council and at this point could start practice as a GP, but most doctors spend an additional few years in various hospital specialties or as trainees in an established practice. After the training period, a doctor often serves as an assistant in a practice before becoming a full partner. At present about 50 percent of medical-school graduates go into general practice.

If the doctor decides to stay in hospital practice, he starts specialty training, spending one year as a senior house officer, two or three years as a registrar and two or three years as a senior registrar. Along the way students take a number of qualifying examinations, usually including those for membership or fellowship in one of the Royal Colleges. If the student stays in the specialist pathway, he must eventually apply for a consultant post and be hired by a regional health authority in order to become a consultant. The basic full-time salary is $15,000 to

$21,000 per year, but after a time the consultant may be considered for merit awards which can double his salary. GPs, in comparison, generally earn $10,000 to $16,000 per year.

In recent years this pattern of education and career development has been questioned by various official committees. A royal commission in 1968 urged that the undergraduate period be used to produce a generally educated person, with a longer period of postgraduate training needed for clinical practice, including general practice. The commission's recommendations produced some experimentation but little substantial change. A recent report from the Royal College of General Practitioners endorsed the recommendation for three years' general professional training for all doctors—including GPs—after registration. Those doctors wishing to specialize in areas other than general practice would then have to take several years of further training.

Critics in Britain point out that these recommendations would increase training to a dysfunctional extent and possibly lead to an increasingly "academic" style of education and practice, with less and less attention to primary medical care. They suggest instead a reduction in academic and specialist training and an emphasis in medical schools on training doctors for primary care. The future course of medical education in Britain is by no means settled.

Remaining Problems

Despite the advances of the past 30 years and the recent reorganization, serious problems remain. One is that of the utilization and cost of drugs. At present in Britain the doctor is free to prescribe any drug—except for "hard drugs of addiction"—at any dose level, for whatever period he chooses. Part of the original assurance given in the formation of the NHS was that doctors would be free to exercise their "clinical judgment" freely. The only check on this freedom is that the number, and cost to the NHS, of all prescriptions written by GPs are monitored, and the practice of those who prescribe at a level considerably higher than the majority of other GPs is reviewed.

Patients pay the chemist 20 pence (about 35 cents) for each prescription filled—on the average, approximately 20 percent of the cost of the drug. The pharmacist is then reimbursed by the NHS for the remainder of the basic cost of the drug plus 25 percent for overhead and profit.

One problem, of course, lies in determining the "cost" of the drug. The pharmaceutical industry, totally in the private sector as in the United States and Sweden but in contrast of course to the situation in the USSR and China, includes the high cost of research and advertising in the price of its drugs. While on the whole there appears to be less spent by the British pharmaceutical industry in advertising and marketing its product than in the United States, the pharmaceutical industry in Britain is still significantly more profitable than British industry as a whole; in the United Kingdom a 14-percent annual return on investment is average for all industry, while the pharmaceutical sector has an average return of 25 percent.

Another unresolved issue is the remaining inequity of distribution—what Dr. John Tudor Hart, a general practitioner and articulate participant-observer in the NHS, calls the "inverse care law: The availability of good medical care tends to vary inversely with the need of the population served." For example, while redistribution of general practitioners from overdoctored areas to underdoctored areas took place in the early years of the National Health Service, the redistribution had practically ceased by 1956, had gone into reverse by 1961, and between 1961 and 1967 the proportion of people in what are defined as "underdoctored" areas rose from 17 percent to 34 percent. Of the 169 new general practitioners who entered practice in underdoctored areas between October 1968 and October 1969, 164 came from other countries.

Furthermore, according to Hart, "In areas with most sickness and death, general practitioners have more work, larger lists, less hospital support and inherit more clinically ineffective traditions of consultation than in the healthiest areas; and hospital doctors shoulder heavier caseloads with less staff and equipment, more obsolete buildings, and suffer recurrent crises in the availability of beds and replacement staff."

That these inequities persist in spite of the development of a universal comprehensive health service and in spite of efforts to redress imbalances in health care between rich and poor raises again the question of whether health care in a society can be altered significantly without radical political, social and economic change as well.

Another critical issue is the distribution of resources within the system. The total expenditures in the hospital sector account for 65 percent of the NHS budget (up from 55 percent in 1950), while general practitioner services account for under 8 percent (down from 11 percent in 1950). There are nine times as many employees in the hospital service as in the community service. This imbalance exists despite the fact that in England and Wales in 1972 there were 6.4 million inpatient admissions and 107.3 million outpatient visits in hospitals, compared with 164.2 million visits to GPs and untold millions of services by the community agencies.

There is, of course, no doubt that even a brief inpatient episode is, by its nature, considerably more expensive than a visit to a GP, and that an outpatient visit also on the average requires more expensive technology and probably more personnel time than a GP visit. Nonetheless the apparent imbalance between the investment and the number of people affected by the services suggests that there are powerful influences—based on the drama and power of technology and of the consultants —which shift allocations toward the hospital sector. And still, despite this apparent imbalance, hospital services are seen as seriously underfunded, with insufficient resources to rebuild and renovate buildings that in many cases are centuries old.

Within the hospital system regional inequities have also been permitted to persist. The London and Liverpool health regions have many more hospital doctors, longer lengths of stay and considerably higher hospital expenditures per person than do regions like Trent in the industrial midlands or more rural East Anglia and Wessex. In short, some of the inequities among regions which existed at the start of the NHS have continued over the 25 years of its life.

Another of the critical problems which remain unsolved by the British health system is the continuing dissatisfaction of many of its physicians. Now that a number of the complaints of the general practitioners have been met, the situation of a few years ago has reversed itself and general practice is increasingly seen by students and doctors as a satisfying career. But among the junior hospital doctors, who are training to become consultants—many of whom will have to wait for years if not forever for one of the limited number of consultant positions, particularly in surgery—there is dissatisfaction and considerable emigration. And even among the prestigious consultants there is at times the pull of extraordinary income or research grants in the United States or other countries more wealthy or more profligate than Britain.

The discontent of the consultants is closely tied to the current controversy over the use of beds in NHS hospitals for the care of private patients. From the start of the health service the labor movement in Britain was deeply opposed to the compromise which permitted private patients to purchase special privileges within the NHS. Moreover, full-time consultants who had been satisfied with their improved status and financial security, as well as other NHS employees, began to resent part-time consultants making extra money from private practice—as the British say, "getting jam to put on their bread and butter." The underlying resentment boiled over when the housekeeping workers at a London teaching hospital refused to serve private patients. All the health-worker trade unions demanded that the government ban private practice from NHS hospitals and a bitter battle has been fought between the Labor government and the leaders of the consultants. The situation is still unresolved, but it appears that the eventual compromise will limit private practice but not abolish it.

As a different aspect of the same controversy about the status of health workers, the Medical Practitioners Union, which had been founded in 1912, in 1970 became a part of a large professional workers union—the Association of Scientific, Technical and Managerial Staffs—with nearly 400,000 members including, for example, laboratory technicians, speech therapists, and pharmacists. Thus a number of doctors perceive themselves as part of a group of workers in health services with common interests and common problems.

With all its remaining problems, Great Britain has nonetheless made an attempt, first in the organization of the National Health Service in 1948 and then in the reorganization of 1974, to set up a rational, integrated system to provide medical care to everyone free of charge at the time of service. There is little doubt that the NHS, at a cost markedly less than that of health services in the United States or Sweden, provides health care and medical care of high technical quality distributed much more equitably than in the Britain of 1948 or in the United States today. Health care and medical care in Britain have, for the most part, been taken out of the marketplace and been made fundamental rights rather than privileges.

4

THE SOVIET UNION—
Centralized
Socialism

The Soviet Union, a centralized society most of whose resources are socialized, has developed a centralized, socialized medical-care system closely linked to the society's structure and goals.

The Setting

The Soviet Union is in land area the largest nation on earth. It covers one-sixth of the earth's surface and extends over almost three times the land area of the contiguous 48 United States. Its population of 255 million, only 20 percent larger than that of the United States, is approximately 60 percent urban and is extremely unevenly distributed; while vast areas are very sparsely populated, the more heavily populated areas have urban and rural population densities as great or greater than those of the United States. The population of the Soviet Union is also diverse ethnically; just over 50 percent are "Russians," while the other 50 percent is composed of over 100 nationality groups such as the Ukrainians, the Uzbeks, the Belorussians, the Tatars and the Kazaks.

The Soviet Union's industrial productivity has risen rapidly over the past 60 years. The Gross National Product per capita in 1975 was $2600; despite its rapid rise, however, it is still considerably lower per capita than that of the United States,

Sweden or Britain. Because its means of industrial production are almost entirely government-owned and -administered, the Soviet Union has far greater control over all of the elements of its economy than does any of the other societies we are discussing. Concomitantly, its planning and management are considerably more centralized than are those of the other countries.

The Soviet Union's health-care system is of interest for several reasons: (1) It provides health care totally free of charge at the time of need to its entire population; (2) it is a government-operated, centrally planned system which functions as an integral part of a planned economy; (3) it has trained vast numbers of physicians (70 percent of whom are women) and other health workers, and consequently has the highest ratio of health workers to population of any country in the world; (4) it has given high priority to services for special problems, such as the prevention of infectious disease and the care of people with medical emergencies; and (5) it has given high priority to services for special groups such as mothers and children and industrial workers, services which in the United States are particularly fragmented and weak.

The Maintenance of Working Capacity

The Fifteenth Congress of the Communist Party of the USSR, which took place in December 1928, marked the beginning of a massive Soviet drive toward economic and military self-sufficiency—in short, a massive drive toward industrialization. The new priority, to make "an unprecedented leap from backwardness to an industrially developed state with a powerful national health system," was accompanied by the slogan: "On from the struggle against epidemics to the fight for more healthy working conditions." Since these first major industrialization efforts of the late 1920s, there has been a heavy emphasis in the Soviet Union on industrial health services. It was clear to the Soviet leaders that high productivity would depend on the good health of industrial workers. Today approximately 30 percent of people of working age receive their health care and medical care through a special network of health services in the industries in which they work.

In factories with 4000 or more workers, industrial medical departments provide a wide range of services including specialist, outpatient and inpatient treatment as well as industrial hygiene. In addition, all coal-mining, oil-refining, oil-extracting, ore-mining and chemical plants with 2000 or more workers are eligible for a department. Between 1950 and 1965 the number of such medical departments in industry nearly doubled.

In hazardous industries, such as the oil and mining industries, a physician's health station is set up if there are over 500 workers. In nonhazardous industries of modest size, and even in relatively small enterprises, there is usually a health station staffed by nonphysician personnel. The number of such health stations in industry more than tripled between 1950 and 1965.

In addition to providing treatment, industrial medical departments are responsible for occupational accidents and diseases, mass screening for tuberculosis and cancer, and the containment of infectious diseases. For example, in 1969 Moscow's Likhachov factory, the largest automobile factory in the USSR, employed 60,000 workers; of these, 600 were medical workers—including 150 doctors—responsible for the provision of medical services at the plant.

The factory had also built its own 1000-bed hospital out of funds from its health-insurance fund. As an example of the Soviet commitment to the "maintenance of working capacity," which is a particularly crucial commitment in a society with a constitutional guarantee of employment, the hospital has special training workshops in which it retrains workers who cannot return to their former jobs because of medical problems.

Health personnel in industry combine clinical medical care —for both work-related and nonwork-related accidents and illness—with preventive medicine. They have responsibility for monitoring the industrial and health environment and, together with outside specialists in occupational hygiene, act as advisers to management. In some instances they also care for employees' families, and in isolated areas or under special conditions they may provide care for the surrounding population as well.

The doctors make routine tours of the workshops and regularly examine the personnel. Workers with chronic illnesses, such as hypertension, diabetes or peptic ulcer, are entitled to thorough checkups twice a year, are eligible for free medication and, if necessary, a special diet subsidized by the trade union. More-specialized care is provided by the general medical network outside the factories.

Workshop doctors, often assisted by volunteers called "health activists," are crucial pivots in the Soviet industrial health system. The doctors are usually occupational-health specialists with an intimate knowledge of their workshops and are responsible for such occupational-health elements as protective clothing, workshop ventilation, dust content and noise levels. "Health activists" play a special role in health education and, among other duties, perform first aid, report on safety hazards, follow up on workers who do not appear for recommended treatment, and visit seriously ill patients at home.

Another significant aspect of Soviet industrial health services are health resorts and sanatoriums, which have been an important element of health care in Russia since the early eighteenth century. By the late 1960s there were over 600 rest homes with about 220,000 places, serving 5 million people a year—all under trade-union auspices.

Finally, of particular interest are the special institutes and hospitals for occupational illnesses in each republic of the USSR. These institutions concentrate patients with occupational disease together with physicians and researchers who have special competence in the field, thereby providing a focus for continued emphasis on occupational health.

There are said to still be great gaps between "theory" and "practice" in occupational health, as in other areas of Soviet society. The problems in industry have been particularly great because of the vast destruction in the most industrialized areas of the USSR during World War II. Massive efforts at rapid postwar reconstruction and the maintenance of obsolete plants have at times led to serious deficiencies in both environmental and occupational health. Indeed, some observers who have studied Soviet factories feel that many are extremely unsanitary and unsafe. Nevertheless, the Soviet Union continues to make a large investment in the maintenance of the working capacity of its industrial workers.

Historical Background

In the tenth century, physicians appeared for the first time in the written records of Kievan Rus, the original Russian state, as attendants to the court and the nobility, but it was not until the nineteenth century that the vast majority of Russian people —the poor who lived in towns and the entire rural population —had anything in the way of medical care aside from folk medicine. There were, of course, earlier hostels and asylums for the indigent sick which were maintained by churches, particularly by monasteries. It is of interest that they were, even at an early time, financed by a special tax which provided limited monies for the care of the poor, for orphans and for the sick.

Employment of physicians by the state—albeit to provide services to a small fraction of the population—became a firmly established tradition as early as the fifteenth century, a tradition that has continued to this day. From the fifteenth to the mid–eighteenth century, physicians were brought to Russia from the West to serve the Czar and the court, and were paid from the public treasury. The country's need for doctors, particularly military surgeons, increased as the army grew during the seventeenth century, and since there were many foreign regiments in the Czar's army who would not fight without surgeons, military surgeons were hired to provide medical and surgical services.

Russia's tradition of centralized medical authority can be traced back to the early seventeenth century when an Apothecary Board was established. Its responsibilities included appointing physicians and surgeons to the army, importing and distributing drugs, examining credentials of foreign physicians who came to work at the court, and, in 1654, establishing a school to train *lekars* (treaters), the Russian equivalent of barber-surgeons. More than a century later, in 1763, after several intervening changes in its name, the board became the Medical Collegium, the direct medical-administrative precursor of the postrevolution People's Commissariat of Health.

The first central effort to strengthen the services provided by local government was the establishment in 1775 of boards of social assistance which were in charge of all charitable and medical institutions. The role of district physician was developed during this period, and in 1797 medical administrations were established in all provincial towns to provide some medical care to the poor.

The Crimean War of the 1850s, between the Russians on one side and the British, French and Ottoman Turks on the other, had dramatic consequences for medical care. For all the countries involved, the great loss of manpower due to illness and the squalid conditions faced by the sick and wounded led to improvements in military medicine (especially by Dr. N. I. Pirogov, a Russian military surgeon who described war as an "epidemic of trauma") and to the development of the profession of nursing and the role of women in it (especially by Florence Nightingale). For the Russians, the military defeat awakened the country and Czar Alexander II to Russia's backwardness in relation to the other European powers. A drive toward modernization led to serious efforts at industrialization, the emancipation in 1861 of the serfs, and the creation in 1864 of the Zemstvo or rural local authority.

The Zemstvo system was designed to decentralize government, to reduce the power of the bureaucracy and to develop limited self-government for a defined district in the countryside. The Zemstvo was a district assembly elected by the inhabitants of the district, but not on the basis of one person, one vote; individual landowners had one-third of the votes, the bourgeoisie one-third, and the peasants one-third. Similar self-government units were simultaneously developed in the towns. Public health services and medical care were provided by local government and were financed by local taxes, with the peasantry— both landowning peasants and landless peasants—bearing more of the tax burden than the nobility.

The living conditions of the peasants were extremely poor, and because of both rural poverty and industrial need there was a substantial migration from the rural to the urban areas, a pattern which was to continue, with interruptions by two major wars, for the next 100 years. Health conditions among the urban workers and the peasants were deplorable; the high illness rates prevalent in "normal times" were compounded by intermittent epidemics and famines which swept through the country.

In the development of medical care Russia had long lagged behind Western Europe. Most physicians practiced in the cities, treating the middle- and upper-class urban population and leaving the care of the peasants and workers to folk healers and to health workers with limited training. Zemstvo medicine was the first attempt to meet Russia's severe health problems, to provide organized medical services to the rural population and to regionalize medical care through the use of defined geographic districts. A significant factor in the nobility's willingness at this particular time to provide medical care to the urban poor and the rural population was a belief, imported from Western Europe, in the theory of infectious disease and the effectiveness of hygiene and medicine in controlling disease. The nobility came to realize that they could not be insulated from the disease around them, that their health was, in part at least, dependent upon the health of all.

The Zemstvos developed two types of health-care systems: a "touring system" in which health personnel traveled around the district from village to village seeing patients, usually on market days; and a "stationary system," which developed through the years, establishing local dispensaries which were supposed to provide basic primary care. In time an increasing number of provinces with densely populated districts adopted the stationary system, while those with sparse population kept the touring system; in many provinces both systems were used, depending on the population density of the district.

In principle the dispensaries, outpatient clinics to which some beds were later added, were to be staffed by district doctors. Specialist care was to be provided in provincial hospitals which were to be staffed by full-time, salaried doctors. But because of the shortage of funds, the Zemstvos were unable to afford doctors, and most of them turned instead to feldshers and midwives. The feldsher, a kind of assistant doctor introduced into his armies by Peter the Great in 1700 as part of his Westernizing efforts, was modeled on the *feldscherer* or "field barber" of the German Army. These health workers, whom we would now think of as army corpsmen, were usually given little more than brief on-the-job training, but were required, in the absence of more formally trained physicians or other personnel, to deal with the entire range of medical-care problems.

The Zemstvos largely used feldshers who were retired after their army service or who were graduates of the large number of feldsher training schools which grew up to meet the Zemstvos' needs. To justify the substitution of feldshers for physicians, the Zemstvos attempted to make a medical-care virtue of their fiscal necessity. An observer at the time reported that the nobility and gentry felt that "the peasant is not accustomed [to] and does not need scientific medical assistance; his diseases are 'simple' and for this a feldsher is enough—a physician treats the masters, and a peasant is treated by a feldsher."

On the positive side, the Zemstvos provided a partial organizational blueprint for the provision of widely accessible medical care, a network of medical stations throughout the country that could be increased and improved, and a tradition of medical care as a public salaried service rather than as a private entrepreneurial enterprise. Zemstvo medicine therefore provided opportunities for idealistic, enthusiastic physicians. One of them was Anton Chekhov, who relied on his experiences in the Zemstvo service for his many stories about rural physicians. Many of the Zemstvo physicians were *Narodniki,* populists who chose the hardship of living in the countryside over the greater comfort of the city in order to be near the people and help to meet their needs. Practice, however, often did not correspond to their lofty ideals.

Starting in 1865 many of the provincial boards of welfare turned their medical facilities over to the Zemstvos, and by 1875 the Zemstvos of the provinces of European Russia had charge of some 300 hospitals and 50 asylums. Since most of these institutions were in appalling condition, one of the first tasks of the Zemstvos was their repair. By 1890, 25 years after the introduction of Zemstvo medicine, 700 new hospitals had been built, mostly in villages, and the 350 district Zemstvos controlled almost 1500 medical stations, 400 dispensaries and 1000 hospitals. Before 1865 there were only 350 physicians working in the rural areas; by 1890 there were almost 2000 physicians and thousands of feldshers providing care to the rural population.

Urban workers were also beneficiaries of medical reforms during the second half of the nineteenth century. In 1866 a law was enacted requiring factory owners to provide medical services for workers and, specifically, one hospital bed for every 100 workers. The law was usually evaded and medical facilities for industrial workers remained grossly inadequate, but the effort was nonetheless a forerunner of the emphasis on industrial health and medical care that was to pervade Soviet medicine in the next century.

By 1892 there were some 12,000 physicians in all of Russia, of whom about one in six was in the service of the Zemstvos. Opportunities had been opened for women to enter medicine; some 500 (1 in 25) of the doctors were women. During this period the medical profession also gained a considerable amount of professional autonomy and political influence. The Pirogov Society of Russian Physicians, named in memory of the surgeon who had distinguished himself in the Crimean War and in other areas of medicine, was founded in 1885. The members, called Pirogovists, were able in spite of czarist autocracy to band together within the liberal tradition of the Russian intelligentsia to campaign actively for specific medical, economic and political reforms. They popularized the idea that many illnesses were "social diseases" that preferentially attacked the poor, and that the only way to deal with such diseases was to eliminate poverty and its attendant social conditions. They even urged the development of state medicine, but insisted on professional autonomy within such a system.

After the overthrow of czarism, under the Kerensky provisional government of February to October 1917, many of these physicians joined in the formation of a Central Medical-Sanitary Council. Its goal was to try to work with the government in the development of a centrally controlled and financed health service. At the same time they protected their right to act individually, in medical and other matters, viewing their professionalism and autonomy as a guarantee both of high standards of medical practice and of their own high social status. Although there is considerable controversy among present-day analysts over its nature and its strength, there was thus at least in some measure a tradition of "liberal" physicians who favored social reform and socially provided rather than entrepreneurially provided medical services; conversely, their insistence on medical autonomy was soon to bring them into conflict with the new Soviet authorities.

Health insurance, which had developed in Germany in 1883 under Bismarck, was spreading to the other European countries. In 1905 a petition that the St. Petersburg workers tried to bring to Czar Nicholas II's Winter Palace—carrying icons and portraits of their czar, their "Little Father," as they marched—had included a demand for social insurance. The czar's troops fired on them and 130 were killed. "Bloody Sunday," as it was called, led to the establishment of a legislative assembly, the Duma.

In 1912, under the influence of the Health Insurance Act introduced in Britain in 1911 by Lloyd George, the Duma passed a social-security law establishing a factory hospital fund financed from contributions from employees and employers.

The fund would provide hospital and outpatient care for workers who suffered work-related accidents or illness, and also pay some other expenses for them and their families. The provisions, however, covered only one-fifth of the total number of workers, and there were no provisions at all for invalids, the elderly or orphans. Furthermore, in practice the law really only covered outpatient services, and even this coverage was discontinued at the time of the outbreak of World War I in 1914.

As Russia entered the war, medical care by fully trained physicians was still a privilege largely confined to the rich and powerful, rural medicine was still in a rudimentary state, the central medical authority barely functioned, and elements of public health were administered by no fewer than 11 government departments. The distinguished medical historian Henry E. Sigerist characterized medical care in pre–World War I Russia as determined by "an economic system that gave wealth to a few and poverty to most, a government system that gave privileges to a few and handicaps to most, a bureaucracy that impeded and obstructed the whole life of the nation—all these factors prevented the people from receiving what medical science could have given them." The crude death rate for the period 1900–14 was about 30 deaths per 1000 population per year. The infant mortality rate during these years was about 250 deaths in the first year of life per 1000 children born alive; in other words, one child in every four failed to survive to its first birthday. Both these figures were approximately double the rates for England and Wales for the same period.

Thus, in 1917 the Bolsheviks inherited a corrupt, economically bankrupt country with major health problems and inadequate medical-care resources. It was a country on the verge of military collapse, weakened and exhausted by epidemics and by lack of food. In 1913 there was, for example, less than 1 reported case of typhus per 1000 population; by 1918 this had risen to 2 cases per 1000; by 1919 to 25 per 1000; and by 1920 to almost 40 cases per 1000. In other words, in 1920, 1 in every 25 people had typhus. It has been estimated that in total some 20 to 30 million people were stricken with the disease and that about 10 percent, which may have amounted to 3 million people or more, died of this disease alone. The number of deaths from 1916 to 1924 from epidemics, it is estimated, reached some 10 million, 7 percent of the population. Lenin is reported to have stated just after the Revolution, "This typhus in a population [already] weakened by hunger and sickness, without bread, soap, fuel, may become such a scourge as not to give us an opportunity to undertake socialist construction. This [must] be the first step in our struggle for culture and for [our] existence."

The Bolsheviks seized power in Petrograd (now Leningrad) during the night of October 25–26, 1917, and on the very next day—one of the ten that "shook the world"—a medical-sanitary committee composed of Bolshevik physicians was formed. At first its mandate was only to organize medical services for the workers and soldiers in the local area, but it was to become the nucleus of the Soviet medical organization at the national level. Because Lenin wanted health care to be, in part, a grass roots movement with the full participation of the people, he advised setting up sections of medicine and public health in the local Councils (Soviets) of Workers' and Peasants' Deputies.

On July 11, 1918, Lenin signed a decree formally establishing the People's Commissariat of Health Protection, whose primary task was to take over the direction of all health-care and medical-care services. Thus, the centralization of these services in a department of cabinet rank was attempted within one year after the seizure of power. For the first time in the history of medicine a single central body was directing—or at least trying to direct—all elements of health- and medical-care work of an entire nation. Dr. Nikolai Alexandrovich Semashko, a close friend, revolutionary ally and former comrade-in-exile of Lenin's, was named the first commissar of health.

Along with the reorganization of medical and health services themselves, social insurance was very much a part of the early revolutionary program. On November 13, 1917, a few days after the Revolution, the Soviet government issued a decree calling for comprehensive health, disability and unemployment insurance. Because of the Civil War and the disorganization that resulted from it, it was not until 1922 that it was possible to establish social insurance in such a large-scale, uniform way, but, in any case, insurance was to be only a transitional phase; by the 1930s a truly comprehensive health service was organized with emphasis on priority for industrial workers, mothers and children.

During this organizational period there was considerable conflict between the medical profession and the Bolshevik leadership. One element of the conflict centered around the Bolsheviks' belief in the importance of making medical service available on a priority basis to those who had received the least medical care prior to the Revolution—the workers, peasants and soldiers. This policy conflicted, the doctors felt, with the "ethical universalism" of medicine, a universalism which the Bolsheviks were quick to point out had not existed prior to the Revolution.

Another critical issue between the physicians and the revolutionary leaders was that of reducing the status of physicians to that of "workers," who with their authority considerably decreased would be considered the equal of other medical workers. The Soviet government felt that the refusal of physicians to cooperate with the new regime was based on the class origins and the class interests of the majority of physicians. Much of the opposition to these issues centered around the Pirogov Society, which was therefore dissolved in 1918.

With foreign intervention and the resumption of hostilities during 1918, the two primary health priorities of the new regime were the provision of medical care for the Red Army and the control of epidemics. Sanitary conditions had worsened, cholera and typhus were rampant, and there was widespread hunger. In 1919 Lenin made his famous statement that "Either the lice defeat socialism or socialism defeats the lice," and the Eighth Party Congress in Moscow set as immediate tasks emphasizing public health; combating social diseases such as tuberculosis, venereal disease and alcoholism; and guaranteeing medical services to all without charge. There was also at this time an early emphasis on maternal and child care; crèches, orphanages and "consultation centers"—outpatient facilities with clinics for mothers and children—were established.

Unfortunately, these efforts were limited by severe shortages of all medical personnel; there were, for example, only 20,000 physicians to serve about 150 million people, 1 for every 7500. In order to train medical personnel as quickly as possible, new medical schools were opened. While indeed attempting to recruit working-class and peasant students, these institutions nonetheless from the very beginning put greater emphasis on academic "merit," and particularly on examination results, than on giving preferential selection on the basis of working-class background.

During the period of the New Economic Policy, from 1921 to 1928, a time of recovery from wars, epidemics, famine and near economic collapse, some concessions were made toward the private sector in medical care. Pharmacies, which had been nationalized in 1918, were returned to their owners, and physicians were permitted to choose between public and private practice. Neither concession was to last long, but during this period it was felt that the public sector was not strong enough single-handedly to provide all the care that was needed.

As the threat of mass epidemics began to subside, the Soviet health authorities turned their attention to medical care for the peasants and for the workers in critical industries. The period from 1928 to 1941 was one of extraordinarily rapid industrialization, collectivization and urbanization. Massive investments in health services, particularly in clinical medicine, accompanied and aided the swift transformation of Soviet society. Health priorities were determined largely by industrial needs and by the dislocation of people that resulted from rapid urbanization. The number of students trained in medical institutes (for physicians) and in middle-medical schools (for nurses, feldshers, pharmacists and midwives) was vastly increased; by 1928 there were three times as many physicians and by 1940 there were seven times as many physicians as there had been in 1917.

During this period of intense, rapid industrialization, the "productive" sectors of the economy were given far higher priority than the "non-productive" service sectors, and women, the last to enter the labor force, become predominant in the "non-productive," less prestigious sectors of the society, such as the health service. By recruiting women into medicine, the Soviets were freeing men for heavy industrial labor. The number of women physicians increased from 10 percent of the total in 1917 to 60 percent in 1940. At the same time the health sector became far more hierarchical, with specialists becoming much more important than generalists, and doctors—specialists and generalists together—becoming far more important than nurses and feldshers. By World War II the system had become both highly centralized and highly stratified.

During World War II the Soviet Union suffered immense losses of medical manpower, facilities and equipment. The loss in population due to the war has been estimated as close to 45 million people, some one-fourth of the total population. Almost 6000 hospitals and clinics were completely destroyed and over 7000 were damaged. Children's institutions and scientific and medical research institutes suffered a similar fate. And yet, because the training of medical personnel was increased during the war, there were more physicians in the Soviet Union in 1946 than before the war. Primary emphasis was given to the care and treatment of sick and wounded soldiers, but special attention was also given to the health of women and the care of their children, since, with the annihilation of vast numbers of working-age males, women now comprised a large part of the civilian labor force. Health authorities, remembering the experience during World War I, feared a recurrence of epidemics, but because of intense antiepidemic work there were none.

Current Organization of Health Care and Medical Care

Today, the USSR has a centrally organized system of health care and medical care provided, with no significant exceptions, totally free of charge at the time of need. Health care services for the community and for the individual; medical care from primary care through superspecialized services, and from tiny rural health stations through huge city hospitals; industrial medicine and occupational-health services; medical research and the education of physicians—all lie within the jurisdiction of the USSR *Ministerstvo Zdravookhranenie*, usually translated as "Ministry of Health" although the Russian title, in use since 1918, may be more literally translated as "Ministry of Health Protection."

Although since the mid-1950s there has been an attempt in the Soviet Union to decentralize some of the administrative apparatus of the health-care system, the system still appears to be strongly oriented toward central direction. The Ministry of Health of the USSR—headed by the minister of health, a "cabinet"-rank member of the Council of Ministers—is responsible for overall direction, planning, supervision and financing of all health- and medical-care services and for establishing norms or standards for the provision of these services to the people. It is also responsible for coordinating medical research, for determining the country's internal need for medical supplies, for determining the amounts of supplies to be produced for export, and for providing technical assistance to the health ministries of the union republics.

The health ministry at the republic level has overall responsibility for planning and operation of health services within its own territory. Below the level of the republic health ministry is the health department of a province or a region. The regional or provincial health department, along with the planning and coordination functions for its area, which it shares with higher levels of the structure, also deals with the day-to-day provision of specific services and directly operates regional health facilities, such as the regional hospital. Attached to each of these departments are specialists (in gynecology, pediatrics, obstetrics and epidemic diseases, for example) who are responsible for the quality of these services within their area.

Municipal and rural health departments, the most local level of health administration, directly finance and supervise the bulk of the health- and medical-care services in the community. They hire and pay health- and medical-care personnel, provide the equipment and facilities with which they work, and are responsible for the health protection and medical care of the people within the area. In the rural areas, however, the rural district hospitals have gradually taken over the functions of the rural health departments and have actually replaced them. Even the "sanitary-epidemiological" control stations of the rural areas have become departments of the rural hospitals.

According to Soviet statistics, by 1974 there were 800,000 "doctors of all qualities in the USSR"; of this number, however, 100,000 were stomatologists (physicians specializing in the oral cavity), who are usually called "dentists" and not included in the category of "physician" in other countries. But even with 700,000 physicians, the USSR has more physicians than any other country, both absolutely and—with one for every 350 people—relative to population size. The doctors are not, however, evenly distributed according to the numbers of the population. Including the stomatologists, they range from one for every 500 people in the Tadzhik SSR to one for every 250 people in the Georgian SSR. Many young physicians are sent to underdoctored areas for three years after the end of their training, but there is considerable resistance on their part to remaining in the rural areas. Rural medical schools are being established as part of the attempt to increase the number of doctors in the rural areas.

Physicians are salaried, as are all health personnel, and there is a distinct hierarchy with large differential increments in pay for length of service and for more specialized or higher administrative positions.

In 1974, 70 percent of all Soviet physicians were women. This is an extraordinarily high percentage compared to other countries, though it actually represents a decline from the 1960s when 74 percent of doctors were women. A large number of these women, however, are in relatively low-status positions; many, for example, are primary-care physicians, who have far less status and income than do the specialists and administrators, who are more often male. Polyclinics, the site of primary care in the cities, have six-and-a-half-hour work shifts, which mesh well with the homemaking role most Soviet women still play. Male physicians often work one and a half or even two shifts, with concomitant higher pay, but such longer hours are frequently impossible for women.

Physicians are trained in medical institutes, operated by the Ministry of Health independently of universities. Places in the institutes are highly sought after, and it is reported that on the average only one in five applicants is admitted; in Moscow and Leningrad there are in some years places for only 10 percent of the applicants. Admission, as we have noted, is said to be based strictly on results of competitive examinations on academic subjects, a method which avoids many of the abuses of admission through favoritism, but which at the same time may prevent the recruitment into medicine of people whose strengths may be other than solely academic and the use of admission into medical education as a means of reducing educational and other inequities within the larger society.

"Middle medical workers" include feldshers, nurses, midwives and pharmacists. Soviet health authorities have had varying views of the feldsher over the years. Shortly after the Revolution, recalcitrant doctors were said to have been in part persuaded to enter salaried service by the threat that they would be replaced by feldshers if they didn't. Very soon, however, the Soviet government decided that the institution of the feldsher should be abandoned; "feldsherism" was considered second-class rural medicine, and the government wanted to equalize care between urban and rural areas.

It was planned that the feldsher was to be upgraded by additional training or replaced by a physician, no new feldsher training schools were to be established, and younger feldshers were to be sent to medical institutes to be trained as physicians, although older feldshers were to be permitted to continue with their work. But the need for health personnel was so great, and the problem of recruiting physicians for the rural areas so difficult, that by the late 1920s and early 1930s the schools for training middle medical workers were increased in number, expanded and reorganized, and resumed their training of feldshers. Feldsher training lagged, however, and still lags, behind the training of physicians and of other middle medical workers, particularly nurses.

Current Soviet writers appear to have two views on the feldsher: On the one hand, they are proud of the overall quality of the training and devotion to duty of the feldsher; on the other they seem concerned about the institution of "feldsherism," especially when the feldsher is described as practicing relatively independently of the physician in rural areas. There is a consistent effort in Soviet writing on the subject to de-emphasize the independent clinical role of the feldsher and to emphasize his role in preventive medicine, his role as an assistant to the physician, and his role as part of a team.

The feldsher holds the place in society of one who graduated from a *technicum*—a secondary vocational school—rather than an institute or university. He is in the position of the technician as compared to the engineer, or the draftsman as compared to the architect. Of course in rural areas where a physician is not available, the feldsher's role and prestige is consequently greater.

Pay scales are tailored to preserve the distinction between the "higher" and the "middle" medical graduate, but the disparity appears to be nowhere near as great as it is in the United States. Reports vary, but the beginning feldsher appears to earn between 70 and 90 percent of the salary of the beginning physician. (Actual salary figures are difficult to interpret because so many services, including rent, are government-subsidized.) The salary is higher, as it also is for physicians, if the feldsher is in a rural area and in a position of greater responsibility—for example, head of a feldsher-midwife station. The feldsher's salary increases with years of experience, and after a few years he is earning more than the initial salary of the physician.

In the hierarchical structure of most Soviet medical institutions the middle medical worker is directly responsible to a physician rather than to other middle medical workers. A similar pattern, of direct responsibility to the physician rather than to a senior feldsher or to another type of middle medical worker, appears to hold for the feldsher. A partial exception to this rule seems to occur in small institutions without physicians, such as the rural feldsher-midwife stations, where the feldsher may be made chief; he still reports directly to a district physician, but he has administrative responsibility for his station and, in part, for the work of the other middle medical workers working with him.

Unlike the Chinese barefoot doctor who is considered a peasant and works as a medical worker part-time and as an agricultural worker part-time, the feldsher is a full-time medical worker who does not consider nonmedical work part of his job. The feldsher's view of how his time should be spent was effectively presented in a 1968 story, "Hay Is Our Main Concern," in *Krokodil,* the Soviet satirical journal. In this story feldshers are required to cut grain to feed their own horses, a task they obviously consider a waste of their time and medical training, as well as—though it is not explicitly stated—below their dignity.

Unlike feldshers, among whom men predominate, nurses are almost all women. There is no problem in recruiting women into nurses' training in the Soviet Union, nor, as in the United States, in keeping them active after marriage and during child rearing. And there is often no separate professional and administrative structure for nurses in hospitals as there is in Sweden, Britain, and the United States. The nurse generally reports directly to the physician; there is usually no direct line of authority between the chief nurse and the staff nurse, and at every level the doctor is in charge.

Mass participation in health care is encouraged through the various levels of government, the trade unions, the Red Cross and the Red Crescent Societies. Active workers in trade unions, factory committees, collective farm associations, and health committees of local soviets are also engaged in health education and preventive medicine.

Urban Health-Care Facilities

Health- and medical-care services at the most basic level differ in the cities and in rural areas. Soviet cities, towns and rural areas are divided into districts, which in turn are divided into microdistricts. A medical district *(rayon)* typically consists of about 40,000 people, and a microdistrict *(uchastok)* of about 4000 people, roughly 3000 adults and 1000 children. A *uchastok* is typically served by two adult-care physicians *(terapevti)* and one pediatrician, plus one or two nurses. People are assigned to health- and medical-care units on the basis of their residence, and boundaries of microdistricts are redrawn periodically to keep pace with population shifts.

As mentioned earlier, urban primary-care services are provided in district polyclinics. In general the adults of the district go to an adult polyclinic and the children to a pediatric polyclinic. No specific method for coordinating the care of a single family is built into the system; indeed, medical-care planners and medical workers in the Soviet Union see no need for coordination of care for the family unit except in cases of certain types of infectious disease. In such cases the coordination is provided by a separate part of the Soviet Health Service, the Sanepid (Sanitary-Epidemiological) Service.

There is great emphasis on seeing the patient in the home. The microdistrict covered by a polyclinic primary-care physician is usually geographically quite small, so that her patients (over 80 percent of primary-care physicians are women) are all located either within walking distance or a relatively short automobile ride from the polyclinic. Generally, all of the adults living within a given apartment building or within an area of a few blocks are patients of the same physician; in fact, records in the polyclinic are filed by address rather than by patient's name. The physician usually spends from one to two hours a day visiting the apartments of patients in her microdistrict.

The hope, of course, is that one doctor will provide continuous medical supervision of the same group of people over a prolonged period of time and that the doctors will become familiar with the area, the patients and the social conditions. Although there is said to be free choice of another physician in the polyclinic, or even in another polyclinic if a patient is dissatisfied, in practice very few patients request transfer to a physician different from the one assigned to the microdistrict in which they live. But problems exist—because of overworked medical personnel, high staff turnover and the difficulty of retaining doctors in primary care. In some polyclinics not all of the positions are filled and some doctors, as noted earlier, work one and a half shifts.

Polyclinics deal with 80–85 percent of all episodes of illness from beginning to end. The adult patient may either first see the primary-care doctor or refer himself to a specialist in the polyclinic; both are considered first-contact physicians. The primary-care doctor may, of course, refer the patient to a polyclinic specialist or, when necessary, directly to a hospital-based specialist. Children's polyclinics are similarly staffed by primary-care pediatricians and pediatric specialists.

Care for patients with chronic illness is provided through special facilities in a process called "dispensarization." There are, for example, dispensaries for cardiovascular disease which serve several polyclinic districts and more specialized ones at the city level. Patients are encouraged to see the specialist regularly—in addition to the general medical care provided at the polyclinic—and all medications prescribed at the dispensaries are provided without cost to the patient. Except for medications for chronic illness, for preventive medicine, and during hospitalization, the patient is required to pay the cost of the medication prescribed; this is, with very few exceptions such as cosmetic surgery, the only payment required from patients.

Along with this so-called open system of medical care, there are a number of special systems. We have already discussed the extensive medical network that serves industrial workers. In addition, there is said to be a "closed" system reserved for members of the Soviet political and cultural elite and their families, and, although they are disparaged as a "remnant of a bourgeois past," there are "paying polyclinics" which provide specialist services for a relatively small fee. These departures from equity appear to be minor, however, compared with the overall thrust toward equity in the entire system.

Primary care in the cities can also be obtained by going directly to the emergency room of a hospital or by telephoning the *Skoraya Pomosch*—the Emergency Medical Service. The call is made simply by dialing 03; from pay telephones, no coins are needed. The call, in the larger cities at least, comes into a central switchboard, is handled by one of a bank of specially trained nonphysician personnel, and may be monitored by a supervising physician or by a feldsher. (During a visit to the Kiev Emergency Medical Service in 1975, U.S. visitors found, probably as a reflection of the rapid increase in the supply of health workers, that all of those handling the calls were feldshers under the supervision of a physician.)

The person taking the call makes a decision among the following alternatives: (1) The caller is asked to go to his or her polyclinic, or, if the call is at night, to go the polyclinic in the morning when it opens; (2) a "medical car" with only a driver and no medical personnel or equipment is dispatched to take the caller to his or her own polyclinic or, if it is closed, to the nearest one that is open; (3) an ambulance with trained personnel and medical equipment is dispatched.

In the large cities, if the decision is that an ambulance is needed, the dispatching personnel have at their disposal specialized ambulances for cardiovascular emergencies (such as heart attacks or strokes) and for trauma (such as an automobile accidents), as well as general ambulances. The specialized ambulances are staffed by specially trained personnel and carry special equipment, which permits diagnosis and stabilization of the patient's condition at the site of the emergency and monitoring for continued stabilization during the trip in the ambulance.

In addition, many of the ambulances, particularly the specialized ones, are equipped with two-way radios for communication with the dispatching station. This permits radio consultation, if needed, on the techniques of stabilization, but that is a relatively infrequent use; more important is the fact that the dispatching station maintains an up-to-the-moment list of available beds at each of the hospitals in the city. Once the nature of the problem is determined at the site, if hospitalization is required the ambulance is directed to the emergency room of the nearest hospital that has an available bed and is equipped for the care of the patient's specific condition.

The system has been highly praised, by visitors from abroad, by Soviet health workers and by the patients themselves, but it is not without its problems. First, it is said to be occasionally delayed in responding, and at times long delayed. Second and probably more important, it is said to be at times inappropriately used for conditions that cannot in any sense be called emergencies or even urgent problems.

The exact magnitude of this problem is difficult to determine, especially since the leaders of the Skoraya take the position that any call to the Skoraya, whatever its nature, is a request for help, and that this in itself makes the call appropriate; less than 1 percent of the calls, they say, are false alarms—that is, malicious mischief. On the other hand, some of the workers in the service indicate that as many as two-thirds of the calls—including those relating to problems such as drunkenness or chronic illness—do not require the specialized service of the Skoraya. In recognition of this problem the *Literaturnaya Gazeta (Literary Gazette),* which despite its name often comments on medical and technical problems, printed an editorial suggesting a fine of seven dollars each time a patient uses the system incorrectly!

Services for "urgent"—as opposed to "emergency"—problems were until recently provided in the cities by the *Neotlozhnaya*. This service was decentralized, based at the district polyclinic, and therefore had access to all of the patient's polyclinic records, making possible a type of care much more closely linked to the patient's preceding and subsequent care. So much confusion existed, however, on the appropriate distinction in the use of the two services that, following a study in Tbilisi, the *Neotlozhnaya* is being eliminated in the big cities and the citizen is now instructed to dial 03 for *any* medical reason after the polyclinic has closed for the day.

In 1974 the Soviet Union reported almost three million hospital beds, or 12 per 1000 people. This contrasts strikingly with its 200,000 beds, or just over 1 per 1000 people, in 1913. Hospitals are regionalized and range in size and service from small inpatient units attached to outpatient clinics, to large district, municipal, regional and specialty hospitals. The specialty hospitals include those for maternal and child care, cardiovascular disease, tuberculosis, cancer and venereal disease.

Until 1974 there was a sharp separation between doctors who worked in the community and those who worked in the hospitals. Because of concern on the part of the Ministry of Health about the isolation of community doctors from hospital practice, health services were reorganized wherever possible in 1974 so that outpatient facilities became formally linked to specific hospitals, and doctors in polyclinics were to work part of their time in hospitals and part in the community. Due to practical problems, the reform did not really take hold, but since then changes have been made which enable community doctors to spend at least part of the year working in the hospital.

Rural Health Services

The organization and provision of primary care in the rural areas of the USSR have been hampered by several factors. A serious problem has been the large differences in population density among the fifteen republics. The Republic of Moldavia, for example, bordering on Rumania, has a population density of 103 persons per square kilometer, while the Republic of Turkmenia on the Caspian Sea has a population density of four persons per square kilometer. Significant differences in resources and wealth also exist among the republics, the least industrialized being the poorest. Finally, the Soviet Union has had major problems persuading doctors to work in rural areas.

Primary care in the rural areas is provided by feldsher-midwife stations. The work of the feldsher-midwife station includes epidemic-control measures; reduction of childhood morbidity and mortality; early case finding, observation and medical service for tuberculosis, malignant tumors and other diseases; provision of "pre-doctor" medical aid to adults and children and of therapeutic procedures prescribed by the doctor; sanitary and hygienic measures to improve the living and working conditions of the people engaged in farm production; and health education. While in the cities the feldsher generally works under the supervision of a physician, in the rural areas he practices relatively independently of the physician except for regular supervisory visits.

Hospital facilities in the rural areas are regionalized and are of three types: intercollective farm hospitals, district hospitals, and regional hospitals. As discussed earlier, the district hospital has increasingly taken over the work of the district health department, with the director of the hospital serving as the district health director. There appears in some instances to have been a consequent shift in priorities from preventive medicine to specialized medical care. This, plus the difficulty in recruiting doctors to serve in the more isolated areas, has at times led to dissatisfaction with care.

Remaining Problems

While the Soviet Union has made a massive and unparalleled commitment to health care and medical care during this century, the current system clearly has its roots in the past. Some aspects of Soviet health care, such as the use of the feldsher and the development of sanatoriums, originated at the time of Peter the Great. Other aspects, such as the use of salaried physicians and reliance on regionalization, stem from the experiments in Zemstvo medicine during the latter part of the nineteenth century.

Nevertheless, perhaps the most significant, far-reaching aspect of the Soviet health-care system has been new—the Soviet government's view since 1917 of health and health care as an integral part of national policy. For over 50 years health care has not been viewed as simply another social service to be provided by a society for its people, but rather as a crucial element in the nation's drive toward becoming a major industrialized collective power. When the priority was rapid industrialization, industrial health was also a priority. When the priority was the maintenance of production during World War II, the workers' health (including women's and therefore children's health) was emphasized. Health has not been seen as an isolated issue but rather as an integral part of the development of the society.

The total integration of health care and medical care with national policy, while positive in many respects, may also have its negative consequences. There is considerable evidence, for example, that the health-care system, particularly the mental-health system, is viewed in part as a political tool of the state to constrain those persons who behave in ways considered inimical to the state.

There are, of course, other serious problems which remain

unsolved in the Soviet health-care system. Despite their vast numbers, maldistribution of health personnel still exists. The Soviet Union, like so many other countries, has not managed to solve the problem of persuading medical personnel, particularly physicians, to work in the rural areas, and consequently there is both a shortage of doctors in the countryside and a rapid turnover of those who do go to work there.

The Soviet Union is also having difficulty keeping physicians in primary care. The lure of specialization, and its greater status and material rewards, frustrates Soviet attempts to provide comprehensive, continuous primary care to the entire population, both urban and rural. Both ambulatory and inpatient care are criticized by various segments of Soviet society. Problems of extreme overcrowding in polyclinics and in hospitals, of doctors spending their time doing paper work rather than seeing and treating patients, and of vast variation in quality are reported both by some Soviet sources and Western reporters.

Because of long waiting periods at times for care, reports repeatedly surface of "black market" payments (either in scarce goods or in money) to workers in the medical-care system. Hedrick Smith, the *New York Times* bureau chief in Moscow for three years, for example, describes instances of such dealings—a workman who paid 50 rubles ($66) to a surgeon to operate on his legs after he fell down an elevator shaft, a chauffeur who paid 150 rubles to have three of his wife's teeth capped, a dentist who smuggled equipment out of his regular clinic in order to set up a thriving private practice.

Severe shortages of drugs and supplies are reported by all sources. Articles in Soviet medical journals and general magazines deplore these shortages and the underlying inefficiency which permits drugs to be available in one city but not in the next. In response to these criticisms the deputy minister of health defends the work of the 24,000 drugstores and more than 93,000 drug-dispensing stations but admits that "requirements for a number of medicinal preparations and medical articles are still not being fully satisfied."

Finally, the Soviet health-care system has by no means solved

—or even, it appears, seriously attacked—the problem of professional dominance, of stratification and hierarchy within the medical profession. The new revolutionary government may have hoped in 1917 and 1918 to change the status of physicians so that they would be considered, and would consider themselves, another group of "workers," and at the same time to reduce the power of physicians over other health workers—but they have not succeeded. The hierarchy among doctors, and among all health personnel, is sharp and clear, and there is no evidence that those currently concerned with health care in the Soviet Union see this hierarchy and elitism as a problem.

Despite these continuing problems, the Soviet Union remains the world's only major power to have made health care and medical care completely free—and largely accessible and equitable—to its people at the time of need. A vast commitment of manpower and other resources was needed to accomplish this herculean task, and the investment has been made.

5

THE PEOPLE'S REPUBLIC OF CHINA— Mass Mobilization

China, a developing socialist society with a unique mix of central planning and local implementation, has developed a medical-care system that stresses self-reliance, popular participation, and decentralization.

The Setting

China's mainland territory, an area almost exactly the same size as the United States, is the home of what is by far the world's largest population, an estimated 850 million people. Of its land area, however, only a relatively small part is arable; China must feed approximately 20 percent of the world's population with only 8 percent of the world's cultivated land.

China's population is, furthermore, most unevenly distributed. The vast majority of the people live in eastern China, with its three great river basins; western China, with its mountains and deserts, is exceedingly sparsely populated. The four least densely populated sections—Inner Mongolia, Sinkiang, Tsinghai and Tibet—comprise just over half of the area of the country, but contain less than 4 percent of the population. In addition, some 80 percent of the Chinese people live in rural areas, an almost exact reverse of the population distribution in

Sweden, Britain and the United States and a far larger proportion of rural population than that of the Soviet Union.

China is still a poor country, technologically far behind the other countries we are discussing. China's GNP per capita is one-thirtieth that of the United States. More specifically, China, with almost four times as many people, produces one-thirtieth the electric power and one-seventh the crude steel produced by the United States. In agriculture, labor-intensive rather than mechanized methods are used.

China's health services have thus had to deal with the needs of a vast country and an even greater population, predominantly rural, unevenly distributed, and extremely poor in material goods compared to the people of the technologically developed countries. But, while statistics are not yet available on the current health status of China's population, visitors in the 1970s reported a nation of healthy-looking, vigorous people. There was no evidence of the malnutrition, ubiquitous infectious disease and other ill health that accompanies poverty in most other countries of the world and was so prevalent in China 30 years ago.

In Shanghai and Peking, China's largest cities, health statistics are now becoming available to Westerners. Data for Shanghai City proper show an infant mortality rate of 12.6 per 1000 live births (comparable to that of Stockholm and far lower than New York City's 18.1 per 1000 for "white" babies and 27.1 per 1000 for "nonwhite" babies) and correspondingly low age-specific death rates at other ages. The life expectancy at birth in Shanghai City proper now appears to be about 70 years, and the leading causes of death are now reported to be cancer, stroke, and heart disease. While Shanghai is not representative of the rest of China, or even of its other large cities, the remarkable changes over the past two decades in Shanghai—the infant mortality rate in 1948 was estimated at 150 per 1000—are probably indicative of rapid changes in health status throughout China.

These changes in health status are certainly not solely the result of changes in medical care or even in health care; improvements in nutrition, sanitation and living standards are at least as important. But changes in health care and in medical care have undoubtedly played an important role. Among those elements of the health- and medical-care system in China that are of special interest to the United States are (1) the society's fundamental redistribution of wealth and power, which makes possible many of the elements in the system; (2) the system's emphasis on preventive medicine; (3) its utilization of traditional Chinese medicine in combination with "Western" medicine; (4) its training of part-time health workers who remain integral members of the community; and (5) its attempts to mobilize the mass of people to protect their own health and the health of their neighbors.

The "Mobilization of the Mass"

At a National Health Conference in Peking in the early 1950s, shortly after the Chinese Communists took power, four principles were adopted which remain the foundation on which medical policy has been structured. While the first three principles are of great importance and will be discussed in detail later in this chapter, we wish to turn first to the fourth: "Health work must be integrated with mass movements." The Chinese leaders recognized well before 1949 that a rapid and dramatic change in the health status of China's vast population could not be imposed from above but was possible only through the full participation of the great mass of its people. "Mobilization of the mass" has been a fundamental ideological principle of Chinese socialism as formulated by Mao Tsetung since the 1920s. The involvement of the population in health problems was therefore an early priority.

Mass participation has taken many forms: People have been educated about the origins of disease and about fundamental principles of prevention; vast numbers of Chinese citizens have participated in defining needs and choosing health personnel and in the Great Patriotic Health Campaigns which emphasize local size sanitation efforts; citizens have been mobilized against specific health hazards such as venereal disease and opium use; and locally based, locally chosen health personnel have been trained to provide first-level medical care and to serve as a link between the population and the medical-care system. "Barefoot doctors" in the rural areas, "street doctors" in the urban neighborhoods and "worker doctors" in the factories remain integrated members of their communities and, as such, provide medical care and activate their neighbors and coworkers around health issues. Furthermore, this "mass mobilization" has been organized and developed within the structure of each community in such a way that the health effort strengthens the community and the community supports the work in health.

Historical Background

There are two distinct streams of medicine in China—"Chinese medicine" and "Western medicine." Until the seventeenth century the history of medicine in China was synonymous with the history of traditional medicine; external influences and invasions of foreigners were simply absorbed and transmitted into the Chinese way of thinking.

Chinese traditional medicine is probably the world's oldest body of medical knowledge, having a history of several thousand years of accumulated empirical observations and abstruse and complex theory. By virtue of its rich and ancient theoretical base, Chinese traditional medicine, which incorporates both diagnosis and therapy, differs from many other systems of folk medicine which are based purely on empirical observations. Diagnostic methods include observation and questioning of the patient, and detailed and prolonged palpation of the pulse; therapy makes use of medicinal herbs, moxibustion, breathing and gymnastic exercises, and acupuncture.

The theoretical concepts of health and disease are based for the most part on a philosophic explanation of nature, on a belief in the unity of man and the universe. It was felt that the human body was constantly influenced by the complementary forces of *yin* and *yang* and that if all of the forces were in perfect order, in harmony with the season and the time of day, the human body would be in good health. If there were any disharmony, disease might result. The Chinese medical system, similar in many ways to the thinking of the ancient Greeks and Arabs and of Europe until the nineteenth century, was based on a belief in the relationship between the macrocosm and the microcosm and in the observation and classification of the properties of natural products.

The traditional medicine that flourished in China led to a wealth of empirical observations. Among them is said to be the discovery of the circulation of the blood almost 2000 years before its discovery in the West. The Chinese discovered the fundamentals of smallpox inoculation (variolation) for the prevention of the more serious, naturally acquired form of the disease in the middle of the sixteenth century; from China the technique was brought by Russian doctors to Turkey, and from there to England and the West. It was not until 1798, over a hundred years later, that Jenner published his observations on cowpox inoculation (vaccination) for the prevention of smallpox.

Physicians were first appointed to the courts of the grandees during the fourth century B.C. The primary responsibility of government physicians attached to the courts was the examination of the numerous personnel of the palace and the early detection of disease; they were also responsible for food control and general hygiene. Thus the Chinese emphasis on prevention is not a purely contemporary phenomenon, for traditionally the physician who knew how to prevent disease was more highly respected than one who waited until the patient was sick.

Under the influence of Taoism, which flourished from the second century to the fifth century after Christ, Chinese physicians continued their emphasis on prevention through their concern with physical exercise, diet and sexual behavior. Moderation in all aspects of living was thought to be essential; thus insufficient activity, for example, was viewed as being as harmful as overexertion. By the end of the Han dynasty in A.D. 220 the Chinese system of traditional medicine was firmly established and in fact was the only medical care of the vast majority of the Chinese people until after Liberation in 1949.

The first Jesuit missionaries began arriving in China at the beginning of the seventeenth century. While this marks the beginning of a new period of medicine in China, penetration of China by Jesuit medicine was limited since most books imported or written by Jesuits in China were not disseminated to Chinese physicians during the Ch'ing dynasty (1644–1912), allegedly, according to one observer, because the Manchu emperor felt the introduction of foreign medicine might "confuse the people."

With the introduction of Western medicine to China, which began in earnest with the missionary efforts of the nineteenth century, there arose great conflicts between the practitioners of the two schools. On the one hand, stories were spread about the "evil practices" of Western doctors; on the other, traditional medicine was condemned as false and superstitious. The Chinese people were often torn between their faith in traditional medicine and the evidence of the efficacy of Western practices, particularly in surgery and obstetrics. In the cities, while the status and prestige of Western doctors increased relative to that of traditional doctors, there were far too few of them to meet the needs of people, particularly the poor. In the rural areas, except for major provincial towns, Western-type medicine was almost nonexistent.

The first American medical missionary to work in China was Peter Parker, a graduate of Yale, who arrived in China in 1834. In 1861 the first Western doctor, William Lockhart, arrived in Peking and became senior physician to the British legation. One month after his arrival in Peking he opened the Peking Hospital of the London Missionary Society. It was an immediate success and treated 22,144 patients during the first year. Lockhart himself described the wide variety of people who used the hospital:

> Persons of all classes, officers of every rank and degree, came and sent their wives, mothers, children and other relatives. Merchants and shopkeepers, working people and villagers, together with numerous beggars, assembled at the hospital. Ladies and respectable women also were present in large numbers, and it was surprising to see the readiness with which they both came for relief and brought their children who were suffering from various diseases.

Schools of Western medicine were established in China during the late nineteenth century and the early decades of the twentieth century. The first was established in Tientsin in 1881 by a Scottish physician, and during the next 30 years several other medical schools were founded under the auspices of foreign governments. Three American universities established medical programs in China during the early part of the twentieth century. A medical school in Hunan province was organized in 1908 as part of the Yale-in-China program, but despite generous funding by Yale and cooperation on the part of the provincial government, the school was closed in 1927 because of growing conflict within China between Chiang Kai-shek and the warlords and xenophobic feeling on the part of the students. The Harvard Medical School of China was opened in Shanghai in 1912 but was closed in 1917 because of financial problems. The University of Pennsylvania sent a team in 1907 to join the medical department of the Canton Christian College.

As part of the Boxer Rebellion and the accompanying hostility toward foreigners, the Peking Hospital was destroyed during the summer of 1900 and more than 100 Protestant missionaries were killed. It became apparent that missionary groups would have to pool their resources; thus in 1906 under the leadership of the London Missionary Society the Union Medical College was founded. Fifteen years later, with funding from the Rockefeller Foundation, it was to become the famed Peking Union Medical College. By 1913 there were, in all,

approximately 500 Chinese students studying Western medicine in China under the auspices of foreign powers and only a
relatively small number of Westerners practicing in China.

The outbreak of pneumonic plague in Manchuria in 1911
significantly advanced the cause of Western medicine in China.
During the five-month duration of the disease 60,000 people
died. Because they did not know how to protect themselves
against the disease, there was a 50-percent mortality rate among
Chinese practitioners of traditional medicine, while among
practitioners of Western medicine there was only a 2-percent
mortality rate. Wu Lien-teh, a Chinese physician who fought
the epidemic, later wrote that this outbreak of plague

> definitely laid the foundation for systematic public health work
> in China. Those in authority from the Emperor downwards,
> who had formerly pledged their faith to old-fashioned medicine,
> now acknowledged that its methods were powerless against
> such severe outbreaks. They were thus compelled to entrust the
> work to modern-trained physicians and to give their consent to
> drastic measures, such as compulsory house-to-house visitation,
> segregation of contacts in camps or wagons, and cremation of
> thousands of corpses which had accumulated at Harbin and
> elsewhere.

During the same period American interest in bringing Western medicine to China sharply increased with the establishment
of the Rockefeller Foundation in 1913. At a conference on
China early in 1914 Charles Eliot, president emeritus of Harvard, expressed the American academic view of practitioners of
traditional Chinese medicine:

> They have no knowledge of the practice of scientific medicine
> and no knowledge of the practice of surgery in the modern
> sense. The Chinese physician uses various drugs and medica-
> ments compounded of strange materials, employs charms and
> incantations, and claims occult powers . . . but of scientific
> diagnosis, major surgery, anesthesia and asepsis he knows noth-
> ing . . . the treatment of disease in the mass of the Chinese
> population is ignorant, superstitious and almost completely in-
> effectual.

President Eliot continued, "We find the gift of Western medicine and surgery to the Oriental populations to be one of the most precious things that Western civilization can do for the East."

Following the conference, the First China Medical Commission recommended, among other activities, the establishment of a "strong" medical school in Peking. The China Medical Board of the Rockefeller Foundation was established to implement this program. The Union Medical College was purchased, and in 1916 the Second China Medical Commission recommended that admission standards to the new medical school, the Peking Union Medical College (PUMC), should closely approximate those of the leading American medical schools. In discussions on whether PUMC should train a relatively few academically excellent physicians who would then become the teachers and leaders of medicine in China, or train a larger number of health workers, the decision was made to train people at the highest level of excellence with a strong emphasis on research.

The desperate need for physicians in China was underscored at the dedication ceremonies in September 1921 by Edward H. Hume, dean of Hunan-Yale, when he cited the statistics on ratios of physicians to population in various countries: In Canada, he said, the ratio was 1 per 1050 population; in Japan, 1 per 1000; in Britain, 1 per 1100; in the United States, 1 per 720 and in China, 1 per 120,000.

Bertrand Russell, however, who visited Peking in 1920 and saw and praised the architecture of the new college, an extremely costly but harmonious blend of the traditional and the utilitarian, was less than totally enthusiastic about the American medical effort:

> Although the educational work of the Americans in China is on the whole admirable, nothing directed by foreigners can adequately satisfy the needs of the country. The Chinese have a civilization and a national temperament in many ways superior to those of white men. A few Europeans ultimately discover this, but Americans never do. They remain always missionaries—not

of Christianity, though they often think that is what they are preaching, but of Americanism.

The Peking Union Medical College was indeed to become a center of excellence in a country racked by poverty, hunger, disease and eventually war. While the teaching and research were distinguished in many departments in both the clinical and basic sciences, the work in public health is particularly noteworthy. John B. Grant, born in China of Canadian parents and educated in Canada and the United States, began to develop a program in public health at PUMC at the time the college was opened. There were essentially no national or municipal public health services in China, and Grant attempted to develop a community-based public health program, establishing an experimental health center in Peking supported jointly by PUMC and the municipality. A program in maternal and child health, which included the training of midwives, operated out of the health center; there was a desperate need for such a program, since, while there were an estimated 200,000 untrained midwives in China during the mid-1920s, there were only 500 trained midwives. A school health program was also developed stressing immunization, sanitation, and health education.

But perhaps the most impressive aspect of Grant's public health work at PUMC was the effort to develop a rural health program in Ting Hsien (county) 100 miles outside of Peking. Village health workers were trained to work with the peasants in the areas of immunization, first aid, the registration of births and deaths, health education and the treatment of minor ailments. A physician was available at a district health station for referrals and the training of the village health workers. While this program was in some ways a forerunner of the present-day Chinese rural health network, it could have little impact because of the political structure of the time and the poverty under which people lived. Nevertheless, some of its elements were nearly 20 years and a revolution ahead of their time for China and untold decades ahead of other developing countries.

With the Japanese occupation in 1941, the PUMC faculty was dispersed to a number of hospitals in the rest of the country. The college reopened in 1947, and was nationalized by the new government on January 20, 1951.

Health Care in China Prior to 1949

There is common agreement that prior to 1949, the date of the formal assumption of state power by Mao Tsetung and the Chinese Communist party—an event the Chinese refer to as the "Liberation"—the state of health of the vast majority of the Chinese people was extremely poor and the health services provided for them were grossly inadequate. The people of China in the 1930s and 1940s suffered the consequences of widespread poverty, poor sanitation, continuing war and rampant disease. The crude death rate was estimated at about 25 deaths per 1000, one of the world's highest. The infant mortality rate was about 200 per 1000 live births; in other words, 1 out of every 5 babies born died in its first year of life.

Most deaths in China were due to infectious diseases, usually complicated by some form of malnutrition. Prevalent infectious diseases included bacterial illnesses such as cholera, diphtheria, gonorrhea, leprosy, meningococcal meningitis, plague, relapsing fever, syphilis, tetanus, tuberculosis, typhoid fever and typhus; viral illnesses such as Japanese B encephalitis, smallpox and trachoma; and parasitic illnesses such as ancylostomiasis (hookworm disease), clonorchiasis, filariasis, kala azar, malaria, paragonimiasis, and schistosomiasis. Venereal disease was widespread. Nutritional illnesses included most known forms of total calorie, protein and specific vitamin deficiencies, including beriberi, pellagra and scurvy. "Malnutrition" was often a euphemism for starvation.

A picture of the health situation in Shanghai, then as now one of the most industrialized cities in China, was given by a Canadian hotel manager who returned to China in 1965 expecting to see the same grim sights he had known for the 20 years prior to 1949:

I searched for scurvy-headed children. Lice-ridden children. Children with inflamed red eyes. Children with bleeding gums. Children with distended stomachs and spindly arms and legs. . . .

I looked for children covered with horrible sores upon which flies feasted. I looked for children having a bowel movement, which, after much strain, would only eject tapeworms.

I looked for child slaves in alleyway factories. Children who worked twelve hours a day, literally chained to small press punches. Children who, if they lost a finger, or worse, often were cast into the streets to beg and forage in garbage bins for future subsistence.

Preventive medicine was almost nonexistent in most of China except for areas where special projects, such as John Grant's work at PUMC, were conducted, usually with foreign funding. Therapeutic medicine of the modern scientific type was almost completely unavailable in the rural areas— where 85 per cent of China's people lived—and for most poor urban dwellers. Estimates of the number of physicians in China in 1949 who were trained in Western medicine vary from 10,000 to 40,000; the best estimate seems to be about 20,000, or approximately one doctor for every 25,000 of the roughly 500 million people in China at that time. Most of these were either doctors from Western countries, usually missionaries, or doctors trained in schools supported and directed from abroad; they were mainly concentrated in the cities of eastern China.

Nurses and other types of health workers were in even shorter supply, and the minimal efforts in the 1930s to train new types of health workers to meet the needs of China's rural population were largely controlled from abroad, usually poorly supported by the people they were supposed to serve and poorly integrated with their lives and needs.

The bulk of the medical care available to the Chinese people was provided by the roughly half-million practitioners of traditional medicine who ranged from poorly educated pill peddlers to well-trained and widely experienced practitioners of the medicine the Chinese had developed over two millennia. These practitioners and those who practiced Western medicine remained deeply mistrustful of each other and blocked each other's efforts in many ways.

Probably most important of all, three-fourths of the Chinese people were said to be illiterate. Cycles of flood and drought kept most of the people starving or, at the least, undernourished. And the limited resources that did exist were maldistributed, so that a few lived in comfort and the vast majority lived a life of grinding poverty. Feelings of powerlessness and hopelessness were widespread; individual efforts were of little avail, and community efforts were almost impossible to organize.

Experiments in meeting these needs were started during the 1930s and 1940s by Mao Tsetung and the People's Liberation Army, first in Kiangsi Province and then, after the Long March, in the areas around Yenan in Shensi Province. These efforts involved mobilizing the people to educate themselves and encouraging them individually and collectively to provide their own health-care and medical-care services.

Health Care From Liberation to the Cultural Revolution

Following Liberation in 1949, the efforts of the 1930s and 1940s to provide health services were expanded into a national policy that included the following elements:

1. Medicine should serve the needs of the workers, peasants and soldiers—that is, those who previously had the least services were now to be the specially favored recipients of services.

2. Preventive medicine should be put first—that is, where resources were limited, preventive medicine was to take precedence over therapeutic medicine.

3. Chinese traditional medicine should be integrated with Western scientific medicine—that is, instead of competing, the practitioners of the two types of medical care should learn from each other.

4. Health work should be conducted with mass participation—that is, everyone in the society was to be encouraged to play an organized role in the protection of his own health and that of his neighbors.

Some of the efforts of the 1950s and early 1960s were based on models from other countries, particularly the Soviet Union, which provided a large amount of technical assistance to China during this period. A number of new medical schools were established, some of the older ones were moved from the cities of the east coast to areas of even greater need further west, and class size was vastly expanded. "Higher" medical education usually consisted of six years, following the completion of some twelve years of previous education, although some schools accepted students with less previous schooling and were said to graduate them after only four or five years of medical education. One school, the China Medical College, located in the buildings of and employing much of the faculty of the former Peking Union Medical College, had an eight-year curriculum and was devoted to the training of teachers and researchers.

These efforts produced a remarkably large number of "higher" medical graduates, including stomatologists, pharmacologists and public-health specialists as well as physicians. It has been estimated that more than 100,000 doctors were trained over 15 years, an increase of some 500 percent. But by 1965 China's population had increased to about 700 million, and the doctor/population ratio was still less than 1 per 5000 people.

At the same time large numbers of "middle" medical schools were established to train assistant doctors (modeled in some ways on the Soviet feldshers), nurses, midwives, pharmacists, technicians and sanitarians. These schools accepted students after nine or ten years of schooling and had a curriculum of two to three years. It has been estimated that some 170,000 assistant doctors, 185,000 nurses, 40,000 midwives and 100,000 pharmacists were trained.

In addition to these efforts to rapidly produce many more professional health workers, people in the community were mobilized to perform health-related tasks themselves. A large-scale attack was made on illiteracy and superstition. By means of mass campaigns, people were organized so as to accomplish together what they could not do individually. One of the best-known of these campaigns (which were often called the Great Patriotic Health Campaigns) was the one aimed at eliminating the "four pests," originally identified as flies, mosquitos, rats and grain-eating sparrows; when the elimination of sparrows appeared likely to produce serious ecological problems, bed-bugs (and in some areas lice or cockroaches) were substituted as targets. People were also encouraged to build sanitation facilities to keep their neighborhoods clean.

Campaigns against specific diseases were also mounted. Thousands of people were trained in short courses to recognize the symptoms and signs of venereal disease, to encourage treatment, and to administer antibiotics when necessary; at the same time the brothels were closed or turned into small factories, and the prostitutes were treated and retrained or sent back to their homes in the countryside. There were also mass campaigns against opium use. Epidemic-prevention centers were established to conduct massive immunization campaigns and to educate people in sanitation and other disease-prevention techniques.

The classic example of the use of mass organization in health was the campaign against schistosomiasis. This campaign was based, according to Joshua Horn, a British surgeon who worked in China for 15 years, on the concept of the "mass line" —"the conviction that the ordinary people possess great strength and wisdom and that when their initiative is given full play they can accomplish miracles." Before the peasants were organized to fight against the snails, they were thoroughly educated in the nature of schistosomiasis by means of lectures, films, posters and radio talks. They were then mobilized twice a year, in March and August, and together with voluntary labor from the People's Liberation Army, students, teachers and office workers, they drained the rivers and ditches, buried the banks of the rivers and smoothed down the buried dirt.

The idea behind the antischistosomiasis program was not only to recruit the people to do the work but also to mobilize their enthusiasm and initiative so that they would fight the disease. The antischistosomiasis effort is particularly illustrative of mass participation, since it mobilized the population in several directions: to move against the snails, to cooperate in case finding and treatment, and to improve environmental sanitation.

In all these health campaigns it was repeatedly stressed that health is important not only for the individual's well-being but also for that of the family, the community and the country as a whole. The basic concept of the mass health campaign is said to be the recognition of a problem important to large numbers of people, the analysis of the problem and recommendation of solutions by technical and political leaders, and then—most important—the thorough discussion of the analysis and recommended solutions with the people so that they can fully accept them as their own.

Using these techniques of mobilizing the general population to participate actively in the provision of medical care and the prevention of illness, such diseases as smallpox, cholera, typhus and plague were completely eliminated. Venereal disease and kala azar were practically eliminated, and diseases such as malaria and filariasis are being rapidly brought under control. Tuberculosis, trachoma, schistosomiasis and ancylostomiasis are still not under full control, although their prevalence is being markedly reduced. In short, the successes in the prevention of infectious disease over a time span of only one generation were truly monumental.

In therapeutic medicine, the campaign to integrate Chinese medicine with Western medicine was designed to (1) make full use of those elements of Chinese medicine that were found effective; (2) provide greater acceptance of Western techniques among those, particularly in the rural areas, who mistrusted them; and (3) efficiently employ the large numbers of practitioners of Chinese medicine. The campaign met with some success, but there was said still to be considerable resistance on both sides. Perhaps of even greater importance, there was said still to be considerable resistance on the part of "higher" medical graduates to practicing in the rural areas where there was the greatest need for them. As a result, by the mid-1960s much of the large rural population still lacked adequate access to medical care.

Health Care Since the Cultural Revolution

In 1965, in a written directive that was one of the forerunners of what came to be known as the Great Proletarian Cultural Revolution, Mao severely criticized the Ministry of Health for what he called its overattention to urban problems. He urged a series of changes in medical education, medical research and medical practice. His statement, known throughout China as the June 26th Directive, concluded: "In medical and health work, put the stress on the rural areas!"

As a result of this directive, and of the Cultural Revolution of 1966–69, much in medicine was markedly reorganized. Higher medical schools began to admit students who had less previous schooling but had the experience of working in factories and in communes; these students were usually selected by the people with whom they had worked and whom they were to return to serve, and in the selection process their ideology was thought to be at least as important as their intellectual ability. The curriculum was restructured to place greater emphasis on practical rather than theoretical aspects, with much more training in traditional Chinese medicine, and was experimentally reduced to about three and a half years instead of six as previously. Medical research in the institutes of the Chinese

Academy of Medical Sciences began to place much greater emphasis on the treatment of common illnesses and especially on the role of Chinese medicine.

The Cultural Revolution also brought about great changes in medical practice. Previously, some mobile health teams had traveled the countryside providing services and training, but now mobile medical teams were organized on a massive scale. Most urban medical workers were required to play a role in these teams or in other work in the rural areas, and a rotation system was organized so that at any given time about one-third of urban health workers were serving outside the cities. They were there not only to provide services for those living in the countryside but also to be themselves "reeducated" by the experience.

Part of their responsibility was the training of large numbers of peasants to provide elements of environmental sanitation, health education, preventive medicine, first aid and primary medical care while continuing their farm work. These peasant health workers came to be known as "barefoot doctors" in the rural areas near Shanghai, where much agricultural work is done barefoot in the rice paddies. Although "barefoot doctors" actually wear shoes most of the time, and especially while performing their medical tasks, the term is used to emphasize the fact that these personnel are peasants who perform their medical work together with their agricultural tasks.

In the area of environmental sanitation, the barefoot doctor has responsibility for, among other things, the proper disposal and later use of human feces as fertilizer, for the purity of drinking water, and for the control of and campaigns against "pests." Many of the sanitation tasks are usually carried out by more junior health aides, whom the barefoot doctor trains and supervises. Immunizations are an important responsibility of the barefoot doctor, but these too are often performed by the health aides, who do their work during lunch hours and "spare time."

Health education and the provision of primary medical care are other important tasks of barefoot doctors. They are also readily available to deal with medical emergencies, since they often work in the fields with their patients and live among them. They are said to be skilled in first aid and in the treatment of "minor and common illnesses." Perhaps most important, their fellow workers know them well and trust them.

The initial training of the barefoot doctors, of whom there are now said to be nearly two million, takes place locally for a period which ranges from three to six months, usually either in the commune or county hospital. Subsequent continuing supervision and training periods are used to improve their knowledge and skills. Barefoot doctors are encouraged to use a wide range of both traditional Chinese and Western medicines, and some have become skilled enough to perform limited forms of major surgery. The complex system of supervision and referral appears to insure that there is generally adequate control of technical quality as well as rational deployment of manpower and access to services.

China's countryside is divided into communes; these are divided into production brigades, which in turn are divided into production teams. The barefoot doctors usually work in health stations at the production brigade level, but do much of their work, both medical and agricultural, with their fellow members of the production team. Their income is generally determined in the same way as that of the other peasants in the commune; each peasant's earnings depend on the total income of the brigade and the number of "work points" that the individual collects. Barefoot doctors receive work points for health work just as they would for agricultural work. They are selected by their fellow peasants for training, and these coworkers often choose the most capable barefoot doctors for education as physicians.

Health workers called "worker doctors" are analogous to the barefoot doctor and work in urban factories. They, too, are selected by their fellow workers and receive short periods of initial training, usually three months. They provide preventive medicine, health education, occupational-health services, first aid and limited primary-care functions on the factory floor or in the factory health center. A system of supervision, continuing education and referral is provided through the doctors and assistant doctors in the factory or in the neighborhood clinic. Worker doctors, like barefoot doctors, perform health work part-time while continuing their other duties, and are paid a salary similar to that of other workers in the factory.

The cities of China are divided into districts of several hundred thousand people; the districts are divided into "neighborhoods" or "streets" of about 50,000 people; the neighborhoods are divided into "residents' committees" or "lanes" of about 2000 people; and the residents' committees into "groups" of about 100 people. Services are decentralized to the lowest level at which they can be given.

Many social services are provided at the group level by elected group leaders and deputy group leaders. Residents' committees usually have health stations which are staffed by "street doctors," another urban counterpart to the barefoot doctor. These workers, formerly "housewives" or retired people, are trained for short periods of time and supervised by the doctors and assistant doctors who work in the clinic or hospital at the neighborhood level; they can refer patients to those facilities or directly to the district general hospital when necessary.

In addition to their health-education and sanitation work, the street doctors, under the supervision of the Department of Public Health of the neighborhood hospital, provide immunizations which are usually given in the residents' committee health station. The street doctors will often go to the homes to bring the children to the health station for immunization, or, if it is necessary for any reason, may give the immunization in the home. The success of their efforts is demonstrated in a number of ways. An immunization chart in a Peking lane health station indicates that about 80 percent of the children had been protected against smallpox (vaccination is not performed if there is any contraindication) and 95 to 100 percent were immunized against tuberculosis (BCG), diphtheria, pertussis, tetanus, poliomyelitis, measles, meningococcal meningitis and Japanese B encephalitis. Charts also document the fall in the incidence of infectious diseases such as measles.

But perhaps the clearest example of the work of the street doctors and their personal and intense involvement with their communities is their work in reducing China's birth rate. Their emphasis is on the importance of family planning in building a new socialist society rather than on the Malthusian concepts of overpopulation leading to poverty and famine. It is recognized in China that birth control, like other facets of human behavior, is intimately tied to one's living conditions and one's level of political consciousness. Therefore family planning, according to Han Suyin, is "based upon the emancipation of the woman, her equality, her right to study and participate in all political decisions, and her heightened social consciousness. Planned parenthood and marriage are factors for the promotion of a socialist society, but they must be based on full equality of both partners, self-respect, and knowledge. It is therefore essential that the masses themselves should grasp all the factors of health work, and themselves carry out the programme."

In the urban lanes, street doctors are responsible for the dissemination of birth control information. They go from door to door, talking with the women about the number of children they want and the birth control methods they are using. By means of monthly visits to the home of each woman of "childbearing age," which is defined as the time of marriage to menopause, street doctors keep careful track of the types of contraceptives used. Most of these workers are housewives, often with two or three children; many have had tubal ligations themselves, so they serve as models for the women they visit. It is said that while no one is "forced" to limit the family to two or three children, great stress is put on educating people on the importance of population control—not necessarily to themselves, but rather to the neighborhood, the city and the nation.

In Shanghai City proper, which probably has the most effective program, the crude birth rate in 1972 was reported to be about 7 per 1000; this, combined with its crude death rate of about 6 per 1000, implies a natural growth rate of only 1 per 1000, or 0.1 percent. Other cities appear to have crude birth rates of between 10 and 20 per 1000; that of Peking City proper, for example, is reported to be 14 per 1000. Many communes have crude birth rates between 15 and 25 per 1000, but communes in outlying and minority-group areas are said to have higher rates; indeed, because of the drastic decline of their numbers prior to Liberation, there is no attempt to encourage birth control among the minority peoples although advice and contraception are available upon request. The overall pattern, however, is a great decline from China's crude birth rate in the 1950s, which is estimated to have been over 40 per 1000.

As noted, almost all the health workers who deal with women around the issue of birth control are women. Indeed women have assumed a large role at all levels of China's medical-care system. It is estimated that approximately 50 percent of the barefoot doctors and the overwhelming majority of street doctors and nurses are women. Some 30 to 40 percent of China's physicians are women, and the percentage is rising since, it is said, approximately 50 percent of medical students are females. Indeed, women seem to be attaining higher positions in medicine than in many other fields.

Marked advances have also been made in the area of hospital care. Hospital facilities in China in 1949 were extraordinarily inadequate; the maximum estimate of the number of hospital beds in 1949 was 90,000, less than one bed per 500 people. Furthermore, hospital beds were concentrated, as were the doctors, in the cities. It has been estimated that some 860 new hospitals averaging 350 beds were built between 1949 and 1957. This amounts to one new hospital completed somewhere in China every three and a half days —a total of some 300,000 beds in eight years. A group of Chinese physicians who visited Canada in 1971 stated that from 1949 to 1965 "the number of hospital beds was increased eightfold," implying that some 400,000 beds were added in the eight years from 1957 to 1965. By June 1965 a Ministry of Health official could proudly state that every county in China had at least one hospital.

Hospitals in the cities range from small neighborhood hospitals, similar to American neighborhood health-care centers, which care only for ambulatory patients, to technologically sophisticated research and teaching hospitals. In Peking, for example, above the neighborhood level there are four research-oriented and specialized hospitals operated under the aegis of the Academy of Medical Services; 23 municipal hospitals, 10 of which have over 500 beds, under the jurisdiction of the Peking Bureau of Public Health; and 20 district hospitals.

The Shoutu (Capital) Hospital, formerly the hospital of the Peking Union Medical College, was called the Fanti (Anti-imperialist) Hospital from the onset of the Cultural Revolution until early 1972 when it was again renamed. The buildings of Peking Union Medical College now have a banner over the main entrance reading *Wei renmin fuwu*—"Serve the People."

Municipal hospitals have jurisdiction over the health services in a given geographical area including those provided by factories, schools, local health stations and district hospitals. They also have responsibility for a segment of the surrounding rural area and send mobile medical teams to the countryside to provide services and train local health workers. This effort was particularly intense during the Cultural Revolution.

In the rural areas many large communes have their own hospital facilities to which patients are referred from the production brigade health station. In the ten rural counties that are part of the Shanghai municipality, for example, there are 212 commune hospitals, with an average of 30 beds each. Commune hospitals are locally administered and financed. County hospitals, which are generally located in the towns and serve the people of the surrounding areas as well as those referred from the communes, are larger and far better equipped than commune hospitals.

Methods of payment for medical care vary widely both in the cities and in the rural areas. An official 1963 Peking publication, *For the Health of the People,* states:

> Free medical care is extended to government employees, industrial workers, miners, university and college students, and to the entire population in some of the national minority areas. To

those who are unable to pay for treatment, the local authorities
. . . grant allowances according to their specific conditions.

Workers in most industries have their medical care paid for by
their factories; their families are subsidized for half the cost of
the services and must pay the balance themselves. Peasants in
many communes may participate in a collective medical-care
system, each family paying into the fund an annual premium
for each of its members. The entire family is then covered for
all medical expenses except for payment of a nominal registration fee.

The Chinese hope to see the elimination of all medical-care
payments "when there are sufficient resources to make this
possible." Apparently this, too, will be done on a decentralized
basis. Meanwhile, the cost of individual services and of prepayment premiums are quite low, even when calculated as a percentage of a Chinese worker's income, and the payments are
therefore felt to be little or no barrier to access to care. On the
other hand, they do make it clear that the resources for medical
care are not unlimited, and that responsibility should be exercised to use them appropriately. The time will come, the Chinese say, when people's socialist consciousness will be raised to
the point where such reminders will no longer be necessary;
that time, despite all the changes, has not yet come.

In summary, the health of the Chinese people has been trans-
formed in just over one generation. This transformation, while
due in large part to the basic changes in the society brought
about by the Revolution, are also due to the nature of the
Chinese health- and medical-care system, whose principles include:

1. A fundamental redistribution of health-care resources
from the service of those who formerly had most to those who
had least. This is being accomplished, especially since the Cultural Revolution, by means of society's full control over health-
care and medical-care resources, with little or none remaining
in the private sector, and by emphasis on narrowing the re-
source gap between the urban and rural areas.

2. A commitment to encouraging the people's own self-reliance and mutual help in meeting health problems. This is being accomplished by mass education, special nationwide campaigns and intensive local neighborhood organization, using techniques that emphasize the importance of health for the family, the community and the nation rather than merely for individual well-being.

3. The training of a large number of full-time professional health workers. This is being accomplished by vastly expanding existing schools, establishing many new ones and, especially since the Cultural Revolution, by exploring techniques for shortening training. But the number of workers who have been trained, though vast, is still insufficient to meet the needs of China's population.

4. The training, more recently, of large numbers of part-time health workers who continue at the same time to be peasants, workers or "housewives." This is being accomplished largely through local initiative but with the cooperation of professional health workers in training, supervision and referral.

5. An emphasis on preventive rather than therapeutic medicine. This is being accomplished by formulating nationwide policies for sanitation, immunization and other preventive measures and then mobilizing for their local implementation.

6. Attempts to preserve and strengthen that which was most valuable in traditional Chinese medicine and using it and its practitioners as a vehicle for the wider distribution of medical care. This is being accomplished by bringing together traditional and modern practitioners in their medical practice and by training each type in the other's techniques.

7. Motivation through fostering a desire for service to others rather than for individual self-aggrandizement. This is being accomplished by widespread campaigns, through every medium of public communication, emphasizing the importance of "serving the people."

Remaining Problems

Despite the vast changes that have taken place in the health of the Chinese people, difficult problems remain to be solved. One decade after Mao Tsetung's severe criticism of the health establishment for focusing on the urban rather than the rural areas, medical care remains considerably more accessible and of higher technical quality in the cities than in the countryside. Buildings, equipment, resources of all kinds are more available in the urban areas. In addition, despite massive training efforts since 1949, a shortage of trained medical personnel still exists, and this shortage is almost surely more pronounced in the countryside than in the cities.

Furthermore, barefoot doctors who have provided a great deal of the medical care in the countryside have been criticized for occasionally attempting to perform more complex tasks than those for which they were trained and have the skills to perform. This is also a consequence of a continuing shortage of trained personnel both to perform complex medical procedures and to supervise lesser-trained workers. Conversely, there are said to be patients who demand a more skilled health worker when one with lesser technical skills could adequately perform the task. In other words, the problem of approximately matching the health worker to the task has still to be fully solved in China, as in all countries.

Problems also remain in the breaking down of hierarchy among medical workers. Attempts to democratize the medical profession have progressed considerably since 1949 and particularly since the Cultural Revolution, but medical decision-making still seems to revolve largely around the physician, whether this is appropriate or not. In addition, the integration of traditional and Western medicine is by no means complete, and thus doctors of traditional medicine probably continue to have less status than "Western"-type doctors.

Many preventable diseases are still present in China in significant numbers, including tuberculosis, trachoma, schistosomiasis and other parasitic and bacterial infections, which indicates that efforts at eradication or control may not be receiving the priority they deserve. Furthermore, cigarette smoking is widespread, particularly among men, and there appears to be little effort to reduce it. The argument is made in China that the rate of lung cancer is quite low, especially compared to China's rates from cancer of the gastrointestinal tract. But since high rates of cigarette smoking may precede the consequent high rates of lung cancer by a decade or more and may also be in part responsible for the rising rate of coronary heart disease, the optimism of China's policy makers in that area may be misplaced.

While the remaining problems should not be minimized, they are small compared to the magnitude of the achievements of the past 25 years and small compared to the demonstrated successes of some of the radical departures from standard methods which the Chinese have introduced. Health care and medical care have been both a reflection of and a leading edge in the restructuring of Chinese society.

Part 3

The Future of Health Care and Medical Care in the United States

6

PAST AND PRESENT

Just as the health-care and medical-care systems of other countries are products of their history and current economic, political, social, and cultural systems, so too is that of the United States. Before we turn to recommendations for the future of our own system, based in part on the perspectives gained by our examination of the systems of other countries, we must briefly review the past history, and the current context, of health care and medical care in the United States.

The Colonial Period

The Puritan immigrants to the colonies brought with them a concept of a static, predetermined and immutable world, one which was determined by God's will. Their purpose was the establishment of a "City of God on Earth." Governor John Winthrop of the Massachusetts Bay Colony, before debarking from his flagship, the Marbella, at Salem on June 12, 1630, wrote a statement of principles for the Puritan Commonwealth in America. Entitled "A Model of Christian Charity," it began: "God Almighty, in His most holy and wise providence, has so disposed of the condition of mankind, as in all times some must be rich; some poor; some high and eminent in power and dignity; others mean and in subjugation."

But God's, and therefore Winthrop's, principles included those of "justice," "mercy" and a strong sense of community. "Every man" was to "afford his help to another in every want or distress." Winthrop urged his followers to

> follow the counsel of Micah: to do justly, to love mercy, to walk humbly with our God. For this end, we must be knit together in this work as one man; we must hold each other in brotherly affection; we must be willing to rid ourselves of our excesses to supply others' necessities; we must uphold a familiar commerce together in all meekness, gentleness, patience, and liberality. We must delight in each other, make others' conditions our own and rejoice together, mourn together, labor and suffer together, always having before our eyes our commission and common work, our community as members of the same body. . . . For we must consider that we shall be like a City upon a Hill; the eyes of all people are on us.

The echoes of this view—at once elitist and idealist, replete with both personal responsibility and the bond of community, continue to reverberate in the land today.

But even then some of the earliest settlers were dissatisfied with the lack of success of the "establishment's" efforts to build a kingdom of heaven on Earth. As early as 1680 religious sects retreated to the wilderness to attempt to establish utopian communities based on harmony, cooperation and a fundamentalist interpretation of the Bible. The religious utopians criticized the immorality of the surrounding society, believed in the perfectibility of human beings through a restructuring of social institutions, and sought to diminish the barriers between man and God, and man and man. Many of the groups owned all property in common and stressed the themes of communal responsibility and mutual aid, themes that were to continue throughout American history as hundreds, perhaps thousands, of utopian communities were organized as alternative communities searching for ways of perfecting life on Earth.

Medical care among the Puritans held few, if any, prospects of cure as we know it, but was based rather on a special kind of preventive approach. It was widely felt that if a person adhered to what Max Weber was later to describe as the "Protestant Ethic"—leading a life compliant with fundamental law, replete with productive works for one's family and community —he would both maintain his covenant with God and achieve health and satisfaction. There were, of course, many remedies used for relief of pain and of some other symptoms of illness, but many of the early Puritan colonists made few major attempts to interfere with what was seen as God's will.

At the same time, in other colonies and in much of New England as well, physicians and surgeons were used much as they had been used in the England from which they came. Captain John Smith provides what is probably the first tribute to an immigrant physician in the New World. Writing of the starvation and sickness at Jamestown, Smith tells of burying by September, 50 of the 105 settlers who had disembarked in May 1607. One group was an exception: "Most of the soldiers," Smith states, "recovered with the skillful diligence of Master Thomas Wolton, our chirurgeon [surgeon] general."

The first settlers and their physicians relied on a post-Renaissance understanding of the world, brought with them from Europe, as the basis for much of their medical care. Native American medical care relied on other theories and was more complex than the European, not only in its pharmacopoeia but also in its methods of controlling what were seen as positive and negative forces in nature and, thereby, controlling these forces in the body. At root, it, like the European system, saw health as a balance of these forces, rather than as an absolute state, and was willing to explore empirically any treatment that changed the balance of forces for the better. The empirical observation by the colonists that many native remedies seemed superior to those brought from Europe may have been responsible for the integration of some of the native herbal medicines into the lives of the new Americans.

In addition both cultures accepted as healers those who could demonstrate healing skills, whatever their training. Spiritual leaders were often seen as having special powers for healing, and in fact there was little separation of roles in social, religious and medical hierarchies. Dr. Thomas Wynne, for example, had practiced medicine in London before coming, with William Penn in 1682, to Pennsylvania, where he combined the practice of medicine with active participation in the Society of Friends and in politics—as a member and speaker of the assembly of the Province of Pennsylvania and one of the justices of the peace for Sussex County. On the other hand, Anne Hutchinson, the dissenting religious leader in Rhode Island, was a practitioner of "general physik," as were many other ministers and their wives.

At times those who were primarily spiritual leaders seemed, in their view of the promotion of health and the care of the sick, far ahead of those whose roles were predominantly those of physicians and surgeons. Following a measles epidemic in Boston in 1713, Cotton Mather published an essay in which he gave an excellent clinical description of the illness and urged: "Before we go any farther, let this Advice for the Sick be principally attended to: Don't kill 'em! That is to say, with mischievous Kindness." Mather had in mind the bloodletting and treatment with strong drugs, especially purgatives, that were common in professional medical practice of the day, for self-limited illnesses like measles as well as for other diseases.

Both the colonists and the native Americans among whom they lived suffered episodes of terrible visitations of disease and death. Boston, for example, suffered five major smallpox epidemics by the start of the eighteenth century, and the sixth, in 1721, was an epidemic in which one in every seven of its inhabitants died. As part of a changing view of what might be done to combat the epidemics, Cotton Mather worked with Dr. Zabdiel Boylston in introduction of "inoculation," immunization through the use of actual smallpox virus obtained from the pustules of people with mild cases rather than vaccination with cowpox virus as is done today.

When Mather tried to have inoculation mandated by law in

Massachusetts, this early "public health" proposal stimulated tremendous controversy. Some of the clergy opposed it as a "distrust of God's overruling care." Some of the doctors opposed it on other grounds. Dr. William Douglass, another Boston physician, strongly pointed out that while those inoculated usually developed only a mild case of smallpox, people in contact with those inoculated could catch virulent and even fatal smallpox from them.

"In short," Douglass wrote to a physician in New York, "I reckon it a sin against society to propagate infection by this means and bring on my neighbor a distemper which might prove fatal and which perhaps he might escape (as many have done) in the ordinary way." Douglass urged further study by qualified physicians, a position that seems at least in part to have been an objection to interference in "professional matters" by laymen.

Despite Mather's considerable influence his proposal was defeated. But inoculation nevertheless spread throughout the colonies, often under legal restrictions that included a minimum quarantine period for those involved. The pattern of use of inoculation differed from that of Britain, where its use was largely restricted to the upper class. Indeed, in 1777, on the recommendation of his physician-in-chief, Washington ordered the inoculation of the Continental Army, the first known instance of an entire army ordered immunized against a communicable disease.

Furthermore, since isolation seemed to offer some protection against the spread of smallpox, whether naturally acquired or acquired by inoculation, and against the spread of other communicable diseases as well, when smallpox and yellow fever threatened New York City in 1738 the city council established a quarantine anchorage off Bedloe's Island and appointed a local doctor to the post of port physician, the city's first health officer.

Thus by the middle of the eighteenth century there were already indications of some of the tensions and contradictions that still pull on the fabric of social life and of medicine in the United States today: "faith" versus "science"; "layman" versus "professional"; "individual" versus "community"; and "private" versus "public." But both in the "established" communities and in the "utopian" ones, a strong tradition of seeking equity and of both self-reliance and mutual aid was established.

The Great Awakening

By the time of the Great Awakening in the colonies, around 1740, there had been a number of cultural changes which allowed the rapid expansion of active social and technical intervention in health problems. The view of nature expanded to one in which the individual could have more influence for change. The universe came to be seen as one in which "all men were created equal"; in which there were natural rights; in which individuals could realize their potential by individual assertion and achievement. The political optimism of the Enlightenment —with its themes of justice, liberty and equality of opportunity —spread over the land and was to find its New World rhetorical expression in the writings of Thomas Paine and in the Declaration of Independence. People also began to accept the notion that one person could help another not only by a common effort but also with a specialized service, and people began to contract with each other to a much greater extent for formal services, including medical care.

As the cities grew, the elementary sanitation measures of the first century of colonization were recognized as inadequate. In the summers of 1741 and 1742 a fever, possibly yellow fever, struck New York City—then consisting of approximately 3000 houses and about 17,000 people. Dr. Cadwallader Colden, in his analysis of the fever, pointed out that it concentrated in the vicinity of the docks, which had been built upon low-lying swamp ground where filth was widespread. He made a series of recommendations for drainage of the swamps and maintenance of sanitation, which until that time had been in private hands.

In response, the city's common council passed a sanitation

ordinance and provided funds for street cleaning, draining and
clearing vacant land, removal of rubbish and garbage, construction and cleaning of privies, and regulation of butchers, slaugh-
terers and tanners. Since dogs and hogs roamed the streets,
ordinances requiring the leashing of dogs and the penning of
hogs were also enacted, but these—like some of the sanitation
ordinances—were largely unenforced. It took 100 years for the
hogs to disappear from the streets of New York City, and the
problem of the dogs is yet to be solved.

The growth of the cities also forced the movement of charity,
which had been largely a private matter, into the public sector.
In 1736 New York City built an almshouse, and in addition to
the support of its port physician, the city council frequently
appropriated funds to employ physicians to care for the destitute sick. Similar actions were taken in other cities, and until
the end of the nineteenth century little distinction was made
between hospitals and almshouses. Even institutions designed
to provide treatment for the "curables" became filled with the
aged poor and the chronically ill.

Folk medicine and self-care remained extremely important.
By the late eighteenth century certain "patent medicines,"
which became easily available and commonly known through
the widespread technology of printing, were sold on a mass
scale in the colonies as well as in England. Manuals for home
use—including the Reverend John Wesley's *Primitive Physic,*
which went through some 30 editions in England and in America—had great public appeal. Since small, isolated settlements
on the frontier could not support a trained doctor, advice on
health care came from itinerant peddlers of nostrums, remedies,
and balsams of life. Most of the doctors were men, but women
could play an important role as healers, and often had a special
role in health care as midwives, since men in some areas were
unavailable or unacceptable for the practice of obstetrics.

The colonies avoided the inheritance of the guild traditions
of England and Scotland which enforced rigid social and professional distinctions among physicians, surgeons and apothecaries. "Physicians" in Britain, most of whom had attained

university degrees and were consequently addressed as "doctor," were the elite among those practicing medicine; they did not, at least in theory, work with their hands as did surgeons, nor engage in trade as did apothecaries. "Surgeons," arising from a tradition of barber-surgeons, were usually trained by apprenticeship; they were addressed, as surgeon Wolton was by John Smith and as surgeons still are in England, simply as "mister." Apothecaries, also trained by apprenticeship, had the task of selling drugs; since they often prescribed them as well, they often took on the role of general practitioners.

While these traditions have continued to play a key role in the organization of medical care in Great Britain (as we saw in Chapter 3), they underwent major modifications when transplanted to the New World. In most of America, as indeed in much of rural England, there was no place for guild distinctions. The few European-university-trained doctors who were available in the colonies were often required to fulfill a wide variety of functions. Most doctors were trained by apprenticeship and practiced general forms of medicine. The apprenticeship system was entirely uncontrolled, and by the mid–eighteenth century in some areas of the colonies the ratio of doctors—or rather, those who called themselves doctors—to population was believed to be extremely high. An estimate for New York City was 1 to 350, and for Williamsburg in 1730 as many as 1 for every 135 people. Thus, although the nature of training and practice was very different and comparisons inexact, there appear to have been considerably higher ratios of doctors to population in parts of the colonies than in the United States today.

Late in the eighteenth century, in the great seaboard cities and even beyond them, physicians trained in European universities began challenging both the prevalent folk medicine and the doctors locally trained by apprenticeship. One early form of challenge was an attempt to create formal legal distinctions; a 1736 Virginia law distinguished between "surgeons and apothecaries who have served an apprenticeship to those trades" and those who had a university degree—the latter being legally permitted to charge twice as much. But success in legal enforcement of professional distinctions—or in public acceptance of them—was rare.

Two other methods were therefore used by the "regulars" to attempt to create professional distinctions between themselves and the "irregulars." The first was the creation of medical schools. Unlike the prevalent British model in which medical schools were built around hospitals, the model followed was that of the university medical schools of continental Europe and of Edinburgh, which was itself an exception to the British model. A group of Edinburgh graduates in 1765 established a medical school in Philadelphia which became part of the University of Pennsylvania 25 years later. This was followed by the formation of the King's College (later Columbia University) Medical School in New York City in 1768 and the Harvard Medical School in Boston in 1783.

The second method was the setting up of local and state medical societies; indeed many of those still in existence originated in the late eighteenth century. These societies became a focus for attempts at formal licensure of the "regular" practitioners, and since almost all of the practitioners—out of necessity or choice—were generalists rather than specialists, the societies, unlike the Royal Colleges of Physicians and of Surgeons in Britain, were largely composed of general physicians.

Those who worked in the medical schools and those who led the medical societies were the elite. Many physicians were also respected community leaders, and indeed several were representatives in the Continental Congresses and signers of the Declaration of Independence. Others, not eligible for these roles because of their social class or race or sex, were nonetheless well-regarded healers. One of the most respected medical men in eighteenth-century Windsor, Connecticut, for example, was said to have been a freed Negro called "Dr. Primus." In New Jersey, medical practice was to a large extent in the hands of women.

At the time of the American Revolution, then, the colonies had some 3500 doctors, about 1 per 1000 people, of whom approximately 400 had medical degrees, and there were few legal distinctions between the "regular" and the "irregular" practitioners. Just about the only model available for organization and payment for medical care as the United States of America came into being was entrepreneurial fee-for-service practice, and little thought was given to medical services either financed or directly provided by local, state or federal government. Indeed, neither public health nor medical care is mentioned in the Constitution, either as powers of the federal government or as powers reserved to the states or to the people.

However, there was already an important exception and precedent in medical care. The Marine Hospital Service, a forerunner of the United States Public Health Service, was formed by Congress in 1798. Its purpose was the care of merchant seamen, who often had difficulty obtaining medical care from local sources in port cities, and it was financed by requiring each ship entering a U.S. port to pay 20 cents per month per seaman.

Thus in both health care and medical care, although the predominant pattern was private, there was early recognition that the public sector had responsibility to meet needs which were not otherwise being met.

Urbanization, Industrialization and the Growth of Medical Institutions

During the seventeenth and eighteenth centuries most people healed or died at home—and were by all accounts much safer there than in the almshouse-hospitals where infectious disease ran rampant. Despite their generally poor image, hospitals specifically for the treatment of the sick were established during the second half of the eighteenth century in Philadelphia, New York and Boston, and began a tradition of training physicians, surgeons and, much later, nurses within the confines of the institution. Many of these early hospitals were formed through the initiative of a group of physicians with the support of wealthy individuals and community groups such as the church.

The current role of the hospital in therapeutic medicine did not fully develop, however, until the late nineteenth century, after the development of anesthesia, improved surgical techniques and other treatment based on a better understanding of human physiology. General acceptance of the idea that some diseases are "caused" by microbes, and widespread belief in the value of antisepsis, came quite late to the United States—not until the last decade of the nineteenth century, some 40 years after its introduction in Europe.

While the academic medical school and the hospital became the dominant sites for medical education and for specialized practice in the port cities of the East Coast, further west the situation was different. During the American westward expansion of the early nineteenth century, large groups of people migrated from the eastern seaboard and from Europe. Opportunities for individuals to function in a variety of roles increased with the formation of new communities, and there was a growing demand for doctors to provide medical services. Much of this demand was met by lay practitioners, frequently women, who usually preferred herbs, diet and caring to the more dangerous—and probably less effective—ministrations of many of the "regular" doctors, who, following the dictates of Benjamin Rush, the most famous physician of the revolutionary period, used massive bloodletting and large doses of laxatives. Indeed Rush warned against "an undue reliance upon the powers of nature in curing disease."

By 1830, 13 states—significantly, not the federal government —had because of pressure from the "regulars" passed medical licensing laws outlawing "irregular" practice and establishing the "regulars" as the only legal healers. This move by the "regulars" may have been premature. There seems to have been little popular support for the idea of a legally defined medical profession, and there developed instead what has been termed the "popular health movement"—an outgrowth of the populist movement. The health care provided by its practitioners is usually now described with epithets of "quackery" and "cultism," but its genesis seems to have been at least in part a reaction against what was seen as a drive for medical "elitism."

Interestingly, the movement's proponents used terms remarkably similar to those used in criticizing doctors in China on the eve of the Great Proletarian Cultural Revolution in 1965. The "regular" doctors were called members of the "parasitic, nonproducing classes," who pandered to the upper class's "lurid taste" for laxatives and bloodletting; the universities that trained them were denounced as places where students "learn to look upon labor as servile and demeaning" and learn to identify with the upper class; "King-craft, Priest-craft, Lawyer-craft and Doctor-craft" were listed at the time as four great evils, what the Chinese today would probably call "four pests."

The peak of the popular health movement also coincided with the beginnings of organized feminism, and the two were closely related. The movement was powerful enough to get medical licensing laws repealed in almost all states, and it was not until the movement degenerated into a group of competing sects that the "regulars" resumed the offensive, in part with the formation of the American Medical Association in 1847. One of the AMA's original announced purposes was that of curtailing "quackery." The battle was to rage in one form or another until the beginning of the twentieth century, when a combination of state medical societies and the AMA finally drove out much "irregular" practice, and with it—until almost the present day—did away with much of the role of women in medicine in the United States.

Physicians of the nineteenth century were viewed, as many physicians had been viewed over the centuries, as experts in both prevention and treatment, and although there was some distinction between these functions in the largest cities, most doctors tried to perform both roles. Unlike Sweden where during the same period salaried health officers worked both in the rural and urban areas, and Britain where medical officers were hired to care for the poor, almost all American practice was private and involved a fee or a payment in kind such as food or clothing for the services rendered. At the same time private physicians performed preventive services and some treatment services for the poor without a fee, establishing a tradition of "charity" medical services in the United States which was prevalent among physicians until the enactment of Medicaid legislation 150 years later. In contrast, as early as 1861 in Russia physicians were hired by the state to deliver personal medical services to people in a defined geographic area and were considered civil servants. Over the next century and a half, this practice spread widely in Europe, but never took root in the United States.

Throughout the century preceding the Industrial Revolution in America, European nations had taken a much greater interest in public health measures, an interest which resulted in early efforts to control communicable disease and even to provide minimum income through social legislation and government action. The United States, however, lagged behind, involved in its own mercantilism and separation from British control; and Americans, having little sense of reliance on a central government, allowed matters of public welfare to languish until poverty and crowding forced them to deal with the issue.

The day of reckoning came with the start of the Industrial Revolution in the mid–nineteenth century. Large numbers of factories were built which spawned surrounding groups of poorly paid, landless workers. Mass migrations of Europeans, especially from Ireland during the early nineteenth century, helped fill the demand for labor in the new factories. The immigrants, poorly educated unskilled laborers in a strange land who performed the most menial jobs for low wages, were prime candidates for the diseases of poverty. The resulting malnutrition and crowding produced the easy mass spread of infectious disease. Death rates in the towns and cities, as in England, grew considerably higher than those in the rural areas.

Devastating epidemics of infectious disease, including typhus and typhoid fevers, yellow fever, smallpox and cholera, at times affected rich and poor alike, however, and therefore aroused much concern. By the mid–nineteenth century it was generally recognized that epidemic diseases were promoted by adverse social conditions, particularly poverty and crowding, but that the wealthy were not immune to them. Thus a large part of the drive for public health measures arose not out of altruism or because the people most afflicted were powerful enough to demand such measures, but because those who did have the power felt themselves endangered by the epidemics of communicable diseases.

As interest was stimulated in disease control in populations, prevention was recognized as possible through sanitation, not merely through the ministrations of individual physicians and surgeons to individual patients. Thus the public health movement in the United States began as a reaction to the effects of poverty and has continued, quite distinct from personal health services, in the areas of sanitation, water supply, and control of communicable diseases.

Another factor in the mid–nineteenth century which had an impact on the nature of both public and personal health services was the beginning of public registration of causes of death in New York and Massachusetts. The practice of public recording of such statistics was a new one at that time in the United States, although it had been done in Europe and Great Britain for several centuries. As early as 1662 John Graunt in England analyzed the Bills of Mortality and began a British tradition of epidemiology, and in 1758 William Farr organized England's vital statistics. A century later in the United States, the initiation of systematic recording and interpretation of statistics brought the alarming infant and maternal mortality rates and the deaths from diseases which were recognized as preventable to the attention of the public.

In 1850 Lemuel Shattuck, a bookseller of Boston and an organizer of the American Statistical Society, was named chairman of a "sanitary survey commission" in Massachusetts. The commission's report outlined the role of polluted waters, bad housing and poor sanitation in causing disease and death, recommended the establishment of a state board of health to correct these conditions, and made 50 specific recommendations for improving sanitation and housing. At almost the same time, John C. Griscom published *The Sanitary Condition of the Laboring Population of New York with Suggestions for Improvements,* describing the dilapidated and overcrowded housing for the steady stream of immigrants pouring into New York City, and relating higher levels of illness and premature death to the conditions under which the poor lived.

Shattuck's and Griscom's reports were a counter to the widespread concept of the "moral inferiority" of the poor, a form of "blaming the victim" of a century ago. The "sanitary reform movement" which developed, in part from these reports, took the view that there was a social responsibility to deal with the environmental conditions that led to ill health.

It took 20 more years, however, for the Massachusetts legislature to actually establish a state board of health—the first in the United States—which, under the chairmanship of Dr. Henry Bowditch, began to try to implement some of these recommendations. In the meantime, despite the recognition that increasing crowding, contaminated water and food, and other consequences of industrialization and urbanization were closely associated with illness and death, morbidity and mortality from these causes continued to increase during the remainder of the nineteenth century.

The Pursuit of Growth, Technology, Power and Wealth

Several major factors coalesced during the post–Civil War period to thrust American medicine toward the technological, cure-oriented, institution-based profession it was to become during the twentieth century: The single-cause theory of disease led to a belief in and search for quick simple cures rather than a community-based, multifaceted approach to care; developments in technology led to increased emphasis on curative medicine rather than public health; large, powerful institutions developed which were to have a major impact on shaping the course of medical care; and attempts to reform medical education led to the ascendancy of the laboratory and the hospital, rather than the home and the doctor's office, in the training of health personnel, and to the consolidation of control of medical education by the university medical schools and by professional organizations.

Before the Civil War there were great controversies about the origins of disease; the speculation revolved mostly around the miasmic theory on the one hand, which attributed epidemics to atmospheric or other general environmental conditions, and, on the other hand, the specific contagion theory, which postulated specific identifiable causes for each disease. In England the two theories were merged, with the understanding that infectious disease arose from a combination of environmental factors, including poverty and malnutrition, and specific contagious factors. The remarkable work of Louis Pasteur and Robert Koch in the identification of specific microbial agents capable of causing disease was interpreted in divergent ways on the two sides of the Atlantic. The theory prevalent in Europe stressed the interplay of many factors, while the specific-agent theory prevailed in the United States. This simplistic notion of a single, specific cause for each disease was to prevail until well into the twentieth century in the United States and had considerable impact on the manner in which medical care developed in this country.

The issue of states' rights was strong in the nineteenth century, and state and local governments, with the specific-agent theory as their major guide, began to feel a responsibility for controlling the spread of bacteria, parasites and other microorganisms; they felt far less obligation, however, to modify the social conditions which promoted this spread of disease. The states assumed responsibility for treatment of mental disease and tuberculosis, and large public hospitals were built by the cities and the states. Management of public water supplies and sewage control were increasingly taken out of the hands of doctors and began to be handled by engineers.

Although the boards of health which were developing in the cities during the pre–Civil War era had an interest in these issues, it was not until after the war that they were given the legal mandate to keep public water supplies clean, to monitor food for contamination and to quarantine victims of infectious diseases, and it was not until 30 years later that health standards were legally required for milk and other foodstuffs. A national board of health was established in 1875, but it was disbanded in 1882 because the idea that public health was not to be considered a responsibility of the federal government continued to be a strong one.

Furthermore, the state boards of health, in attempting to correct some of the more flagrant threats to health, ran into the laissez-faire philosophy that dominated the judicial system of the time. The New York State legislature in 1884 enacted a law which attempted to prohibit as a health measure the manufacture of cigars in tiny, airless tenement rooms which also served as the living quarters for the cigar workers. One Peter Jacobs owned such a tenement factory, keeping his tenants in an economic vise by collecting high rents and paying low wages for the work. His appeal from his conviction under the new law was upheld in 1885 by the New York State Court of Appeals: ". . . this law interferes with the profitable and free use of his property by the owner . . . and trammels him in the application of his industry and the disposition of his labor, and thus . . . arbitrarily deprives him of his property and of some portion of his personal liberty."

As in politics, education and industry, issues of power and control of resources became significant in late-nineteenth-century development of medical care. The end of the nineteenth century and the start of the twentieth also brought the beginning of the explosion of science and technology in medicine. Together these developments led to concentration of power in medical schools and, later, in research institutes and teaching hospitals. The prototype of the twentieth-century pattern for medical schools was the Johns Hopkins Medical School, formed during the 1890s as an attempt to concentrate power and resources around the most advanced knowledge of European universities and skills developed in the United States.

At the same time, members of the teaching faculties of Johns Hopkins and other leading medical schools became a powerful force within the American Medical Association, which had been from the time of its formation in 1847 until the turn of the century a rather loosely structured organization, mainly concerned with the protection and continuing education of its members. In 1901 there was a major reorganization of the AMA. Councils were developed, including one on medical education, and during the first decade of the century, as the organization was developing a strong leadership and a large following, it began to take positions on social issues.

By 1910 the AMA was concerned with the issue of financing national health insurance, and in a well-publicized statement it indicated that the medical profession had a "responsibility to society . . . and must change for its betterment." In 1916 the AMA's committee on social insurance recommended a system of national health insurance. Over a period of 20 years the AMA had come to recognize the need for coordination and equitable distribution of medical services within society. In this and in other ways a segment of pre–World War I organized medicine in the United States seemed, like the Pirogovists in Russia and the members of the Medical Practitioners Union in Britain, to advocate liberal reform of the health-care and medical-care system.

Science, meanwhile, had provided a new vocabulary for the university; and the use of anesthetics, combined with an understanding, in later decades, of specific methods of treatment such as insulin, antibiotics, cortisone and tranquilizers, allowed the development of a power base of persons who could perform services seen as efficacious. The emphasis on the utilization of scientific theory in medical care, especially in a society wedded to the single-agent theory of the genesis of illness, developed into a focus on disease itself rather than on therapy, prevention of disability, and caring for the "whole person." The old-fashioned family doctor had viewed patients in relation to their families and communities and had apparently been able to some extent to help people cope with problems of personal life, family and society; the vigor with which American medicine adopted a "scientific" approach left many of these other functions in the lurch. Science allowed the physician to deal with tissues and organs, which were far easier to comprehend than were the dynamics of human relationships or the complexities of disease prevention. Many physicians made efforts to integrate the various roles, but the major thrust was toward medical science.

There were other changes in American society which had an impact on the nature of modern medical services. Until the turn of the century, medical care had been relatively simple and inexpensive, even for the poor. But starting in the early twentieth century, medical care became significantly more complex and expensive. At the same time, the urban poor grew vastly in numbers, both as a result of immigration from Europe and migration from rural areas, and the demand for health services for the poor increased. Academic medicine had a use for such people in its teaching and research activities, and in fact the poor in many cases received advanced, specialized medical care on the basis that treatment of charity cases was a contribution to medical education.

In addition to the expanded development of publicly supported general hospitals, local governments for the first time became involved in the delivery of specialized personal health services outside the hospital. During the first decade of the twentieth century, New York and later other large cities allowed their boards of health to take a special interest in maternal and child health care at public expense. Efforts were organized around the requirements for milk and the development of other nutritional programs for children, especially within the public school system. Public education became almost universal and then mandatory, and there was a new effort to educate children who were handicapped physically or mentally.

Lillian Wald, the founder in 1893 of the Henry Street Settlement on the Lower East Side of New York City, established the world's first public health nursing service to provide instruction about health care and sanitation in the home. She also fought for a government agency devoted to the health and safety of children and was one of the organizers of a school nursing system. Later, school systems around the country were increasingly required to provide medical services for children who were not otherwise receiving them, including children with remediable deficiencies such as poor vision and hearing.

Thus began a new era of medical intervention in public institutions, which later developed in some instances into attempts to provide comprehensive care.

During the late nineteenth century as many as 400 medical schools were founded in the United States. Most lasted only a short time, but some 150 medical schools were operating near the end of the century. Most of these were privately owned institutions, lacked standardized requirements and produced physicians and surgeons who had inconsistent and often inadequate education. Some medical students were indeed trained in European-style schools that offered a combination of humanitarianism and utilization of the new knowledge of the nature and treatment of disease; others were trained in schools that, by any standards, could only produce charlatans.

The Carnegie Commission therefore authorized Abraham Flexner, a nonphysician, to evaluate medical education throughout the country. In 1910 the "Flexner Report" disclosed many of the inadequacies in medical education and, within a few years, brought about the closing of many of the "borderline" medical schools. There is little doubt that many of these schools required closing for the protection of the public from their graduates. But Flexner's advice also had other far-reaching consequences.

The adoption of the report's recommendations helped further the ascendancy of large medical institutions, such as teaching hospitals and medical schools with their emphasis on science and technology and their de-emphasis of caring. It also signaled the emerging power of the huge foundations, which have continued to exert a powerful influence on American medicine, particularly in its educational and research priorities. This influence has been wielded by "well-meaning" and often "liberal" foundation staffs and boards and indeed has led to a number of experiments in the provision of medical care, but its overall impact has been to make medicine more responsive to private pressures and less responsible to public control.

Finally, the closing of many medical schools in the wake of the Flexner report markedly cut the production of physicians, leading to a seller's market in medicine which has continued to the present time.

The profound changes in attitude which followed World War I—the shift in U.S. public opinion toward isolationism, protectionism and various forms of escapism—were reflected within organized medicine. In the early 1920s the AMA was taken over by a group of private practitioners with a very different philosophy from that of the academics who had espoused national health insurance earlier in the century, and the organization began to function as a much more clearly defined special-interest group. By discouraging any expansion of medical education, it effectively restricted the numbers of physicians delivering medical services, a restriction that had no discernible relationship to health-care needs and seemed to be based almost entirely on protectionism. The AMA during this period also began to oppose any effective system of national health insurance—with its attendant controls over utilization of services and fees—a stand that has continued to this day.

Thus, during the 50 years ending with the 1920s the pursuit of property, with its philosophy of laissez-faire and its spawning of huge corporations, made the protection of health increasingly difficult despite the growing recognition that the poverty and pollution on which the wealth was based were destructive to health. It appeared for a time that organized medicine would place itself at least to some extent on the side of the exploited, but technological, educational and social changes rapidly altered the nature of the profession and it became as monopolistic and self-serving in the pursuit of wealth and power as the institutions which surrounded and shaped it.

Changes Brought by the Depression and World War II

With the onset of the Depression there came a recognition that the pursuit of wealth by some would not produce even a minimum standard of living for many, not to speak of equity. The United States, to protect its monied class against more fundamental change, attempted to provide social insurance ("social security") benefits, unemployment income, federally funded job opportunities and, to a certain extent, welfare or "charity" benefits to those with special needs. But it still did not move toward providing broad-based specific support of medical care, as several other industrialized countries already had.

Nonetheless, the social security legislation of the 1930s was of great importance in that it embodied a shift from local control of social welfare to more centralized control. The cost of caring for children and the elderly, and to an increasing extent the jobless, the homeless and the poor, came to be perceived by the people as part of the nation's, or at least the individual state's, collective responsibility. But in medicine as in the society as a whole, just enough reforms were introduced to keep any kind of fundamental change in distribution of power or resources from occurring.

The situation in medicine was summarized in 1932 by the distinguished Committee on the Costs of Medical Care, a description that would be hard to improve on today:

> The problem of providing satisfactory medical service to all the people of the United States at costs they can meet is a pressing one. At the present time many persons do not receive service which is adequate in either quantity or quality and the costs of service are inequitably distributed. . . . Furthermore, these con-

ditions are . . . largely unnecessary. The United States has the
economic resources, the organizing ability and the technical
experience to solve this problem.

The federal government did enter the field of medical care in
a number of ways. The Federal Emergency Relief Administration, created in 1933 to assist states in maintaining their programs for unemployment and other relief, also provided
medical care and supplies to recipients of unemployment relief
and helped to make the public aware of the inadequacy of
existing health facilities, especially in the rural areas. The Social
Security Act of 1935, along with its better-known function of
provision of income for the elderly, authorized grants to states
for maternal and child health and welfare programs and authorized appropriations to assist states in organizing and maintaining more adequate state and local services. Workmen's
compensation insurance for work-related injuries was federally
mandated. And in 1939 the Wagner-Murray-Dingell bill to
create a system of compulsory national health insurance for
employees and their dependents was first proposed, but, needless to say, was not enacted.

In the private sector, the 1930s was the period during which
commercial insurance plans slowly gained favor with organized
medicine. In 1933 the American Hospital Association endorsed
hospital prepayment insurance plans and the AMA House of
Delegates supported voluntary insurance under medical control. In 1934 private insurance companies first offered commercial insurance against the costs of hospitalization, and in 1935
the AMA House of Delegates approved in principle tax-supported medical care for the "indigent," coupled with voluntary
health insurance for those above the level of indigence.

In addition, labor unions began to demand health insurance
as an element in collective bargaining with employers. In 1943
the International Ladies Garment Workers Union succeeded in
obtaining for some of their workers in Philadelphia the first
medical benefits provided under collective bargaining other
than weekly sick benefits, and in 1947 medical services were

first provided directly to paraplegic miners under the United Mine Workers Welfare and Retirement Fund.

In the early 1940s the Blue Cross and Blue Shield plans were developed in each state, largely supported by and controlled by physicians and hospital administrators who, as costs of medical care began to escalate, recognized the importance of these plans both to themselves and to their patients. These forms of insurance covered many hospital and surgical costs, but the cost of drugs, out-of-hospital care, dental care and other services were usually excluded. Furthermore, these plans were only available to those who could pay for them or those whose employers could bear the costs; the poor continued to depend on "welfare" institutions.

During World War II, major construction projects were begun in isolated areas of the western United States where workers and their families had no access to medical services. A medical-care system was formed specifically for the care of some of these workers, and the costs were contracted for on a yearly basis. The Kaiser-Permanente Medical Care Program has expanded enormously since then and is now the largest private prepaid group practice of medical care in the United States. It currently enrolls over three million people for whom it provides specified health-care and medical-care service at monthly prepaid rates, contracted for either individually or through groups such as employers.

A cooperative effort was seen by many as necessary for recovery from the effects of the Depression and, later, for national defense during the rapid rise of fascism in Europe. Seeds were being sown for the use of health insurance and health services as part of a process of a more just distribution of society's resources. The introduction of hospitalization insurance, the postwar explosion in medical technology, and the gross maldistribution of hospital beds led Congress to authorize federal funding of hospital construction through the Hill-Burton law. This provided a further stimulus to make hospitals the focus for the development of medical care.

The postwar role of the federal government in the direct provision of medical care also expanded rapidly through the

Veterans Administration's assumption of responsibility for the medical care of millions of ex-servicemen, along with the armed forces' continued provision of medical care for those in the military and some of their dependents. It has been estimated that some 85 percent of the Veterans Administration's medical-care activities are now concerned with disease and disability that are not service-related. The federal government's direct role in medical care has also included the Public Health Service's maintenance of five hospitals and some twenty clinics for merchant seamen, a leprosarium, a hospital for patients suffering from drug addiction, the Indian Health Service, and health services for isolated areas of Alaska. In 1953 the establishment of the Department of Health, Education and Welfare as a cabinet-level department within the administrative branch of the government created a legitimate forum for further promotion and development of the federal government's role in health. It also coincided with a vast expansion in the resources made available to research through the National Institutes of Health.

With all these shifts, however, the fundamental control over health care—as over most aspects of society's goods and services—remained in private hands. Even many of those services which were financed by government or were otherwise "public" in nature were largely controlled by entrepreneurs and corporations of the private sector. The stage was thus set, as funds became increasingly available, for uncontrolled, uncoordinated, chaotic technological and institutional growth.

The Expansion of the Public Sector During the 1960s

The opportunity for massive growth of federal involvement in medical care came with the election of the Johnson-landslide Democratic Congress of 1964 after the assassination of John Kennedy in 1963. During the administrations of Truman, Eisenhower and Kennedy, there had been abortive attempts to develop national health-insurance coverage for all Americans, but major health-insurance legislation was not enacted until the burst of social legislation of the Eighty-ninth Congress. The struggles between the various factions—those who wanted health insurance to be a form of social insurance for all as a matter of right and those who wanted it to be a form of welfare for those who could pass a means test; those who wanted it to be federally administered and those who wanted it to be locally administered; those who wanted universal coverage and those who wanted coverage of specific groups of people at special risk —resulted in an unlikely compromise: Two specific programs were enacted as amendments to the Social Security Act.

One, Medicare, was an expansion of the social security system to provide coverage for the cost of health services for essentially everyone over the age of 65 and was largely federally administered. The other, Medicaid, was a form of welfare for the "medically indigent" and was designed and administered on a state-by-state basis with federal matching funds. Together these programs indeed provided funding for large amounts of medical care to those who had previously been financially unable to obtain it, but, as we have explored in Chapter 1, they also led to enormous escalation in costs, uncontrolled growth of institutions and technology, and enormous incomes and profits for specific elements in the system. State control of Medicaid led to enormous inequalities in programs among states. There was also the incentive, because of the structure of Medicaid and to a certain extent of Medicare, for deception and fraud, both by patients and by medical-care providers. Overall, the insurance companies which were permitted to play a role in the administration of the programs, and the doctors and medical institutions who are paid by them, are among the greatest beneficiaries.

Duplication and lack of coordination of medical services were also recognized as special problems during the 1960s. The same Congress that enacted Medicare and Medicaid enacted Comprehensive Health Planning legislation and Regional Medical Program legislation (more popularly known as the "Heart Disease, Cancer and Stroke Program") in an attempt to ratio-

nalize and decentralize health-care planning and to expand the
base of knowledge and narrow the gap between knowledge and
practice for specific illnesses which are the leading causes of
death—but, significantly, not the leading causes of disability—
in the United States. Due to the unwillingness of the medical
profession and of medical-care institutions to permit control
over their activities, these programs had little power and little
significant impact, and were to last only a short time.

Perhaps of greatest long-term significance was the emergence
during the 1960s of human-rights movements—for blacks, for
women and for other groups which have been discriminated
against in American society. These movements, in part efforts
to establish as rights certain services that had previously been
seen as privileges, played an important role both in health care
and in medical care in the United States in the 1960s. The
federal government's newly established Office of Economic Opportunity funded neighborhood medical-care demonstration
projects in poor urban and rural areas, the goal being the provision of comprehensive and integrated medical services to those
who were otherwise without access to them. Other centers were
started by the Children's Bureau and by the Department of
Health, Education and Welfare.

Although these demonstration health centers were to be deci-
mated in a few years by the advent of the Nixon administration,
they provided models for new ways to deal with health care.
The Martin Luther King Health Center in the South Bronx
developed a program for the training and integration of local
people into a health team of family health workers. The Mound
Bayou Health Center in the delta area of Mississippi combined
health care with agricultural and community development.
When patients were seen with symptoms of malnutrition, prescriptions were written for the specific treatment for malnutrition—adequate amounts and types of food—and the cost was
paid from the medical center's funds.

Methods for providing comprehensive, integrated, continuing, family-centered personal services were developed and implemented—for people who were accustomed only to

fragmented, episodic, impersonal care. These models were expensive but they showed it could be done, and reductions in missed-appointment rates, hospitalization rates and infant mortality rates testified to their effectiveness.

In sum, the 1960s saw attempts by the federal government to meet some of the problems of inaccessibility of medical care to the poor, of the high out-of-pocket cost of medical care to the aged, and of the fragmentation and duplication of medical services. But the efforts were themselves fragmented and often in conflict with one another, and these contradictions—together with the fact that the war on poverty soon took a clear second place to the war in Vietnam—led, as we have seen, to a worsening of some of the very problems they were designed to ameliorate.

The Partial Dismantling of the Public Medical-Care System During the 1970s

Over the past decade not only has the U.S. health- and medical-care system not been mobilized to meet societal needs but it has in many ways been seriously weakened. In particular the Nixon-Ford years saw a partial dismantling of public medical care in favor of private medical care, and a relative reduction in federal funding for services for the poor and for minority groups. The destruction was heralded by a report issued by the Department of Health, Education and Welfare six months after President Nixon's inauguration. It is of interest that this report was presented by President Nixon at a press conference in which he warned of a "massive crisis" and an imminent "breakdown" of the medical-care system. His solution, a major recommendation of the report, was: "Much of the burden must be taken up by the private sector since it has the primary responsibility for the delivery of health care."

Over the next eight years, with accelerating speed, the Nixon, and then the Ford, administration did precisely what it had promised to do. In the name of "efficiency," "economy" and "local initiative," it sought to weaken medical care provided through public funds relative to privately paid-for medical care. In so doing, it attempted to destroy precisely those parts of the American health-care system that, however inadequately, provide most of the service available to the poor, the mentally ill, the chronically ill, the elderly—in sum, the people least able to purchase adequate medical care at inflated prices in the private market.

In the 1960s there had been some attempt to provide health services to those who most needed them. Programs—inadequate programs, but nonetheless some programs—for specific categorical health-care needs had been developed. Funds—inadequate funds, but nonetheless some funds—for initial training of health workers of all types and for continued training of those already working had been available.

Under the Nixon administration, however, resources for the education of physicians and other health workers were seriously weakened, and there were dysfunctional shifts and cuts in research priorities. At the same time, the administration sought to give private-sector providers, such as insurance companies and the private practitioners represented by the American Medical Association, precisely what they had been asking for—a monopoly in private hands on the provision of health care in the United States. During this period, not surprisingly, the two-class system which characterizes much of U.S. medicine grew even more widely disparate in its care for the affluent and for the poor, as exemplified by Medicaid mills and desperately underfunded municipal health-care and medical-care facilities. At the same time, all groups have seen their out-of-pocket health-care costs rise, with no significant improvement in the distribution or quality of care.

The wanton destruction of some of the best efforts of the past decade to provide public medical care for those who need it most did not serve the high-sounding goals of "economy," "efficiency" or "local initiative." The decimation of public services in health care was part of a process which affected education, housing, transportation and other services in much the same way, and served other goals—the goals of those whom the administration saw as its supporters. This constituency included, on the one hand, the private practitioners of the American Medical Association, other private providers and insurers, and the large foundations and medical institutions, all of whom dominate American medicine; and on the other hand, those well-enough-off to be able to purchase their medical care in an inflated private market and who view tax-supported medical care as an imposition on them. This was political use of health services in its most blatant form.

Meanwhile, the liberal solutions offered by Democrats, like Edward Kennedy in the Senate and Paul Rogers in the House, while clearly more responsive to people's needs for care and to some of the issues of equity and community, also did not come to grips with the overall problems in a unified way. In 1971 the continued shortage of medical care, particularly in certain rural areas, led to the development of a National Health Service Corps as a part of the U.S. Public Health Service. The effort was small compared to the magnitude of the problem, but several hundred communities that previously had no physicians, or clearly too few to meet their needs, at least had some physicians assigned for a period. Although it is too soon to judge the overall results, it appears that very few of these physicians stayed very long beyond their assigned periods and few accomplished any lasting change in medical care in the communities to which they were assigned. A host of other separate bills attempted to deal with fragments of the health- and medical-care system such as the training of health personnel, specific diseases such as diabetes and arthritis, and the control of toxic substances.

The only attempt of any breadth to deal with planning the medical-care system was a bill enacted over the opposition of the Nixon and Ford administrations in 1974. In view of the recognized failure of the Hill-Burton Hospital Construction Program, the Comprehensive Health Planning Agencies and the Regional Medical Programs (Heart Disease, Cancer and Stroke), all these programs were replaced by a much broader form of health-planning legislation—the Health Planning and Resources Development Act, which set up Health Systems Agencies across the nation. This program is likely to have considerably more impact on the planning and development of health facilities and services financed by federal funds, but relatively little impact on other parts of the health-care system. In any event, despite its emphasis on "consumer" representation, it is largely dominated by the forces which have historically dominated medical-care policy in the United States. Where consumers play a significant role, they almost invariably represent no clear constituency to which they are accountable, and therefore often make decisions on the basis of private agendas rather than community goals.

During the 1970s both the Democratic Congress and the Republican administration committed themselves to the attempt to control costs, and legislation was enacted in an effort to monitor the utilization of services. Organized medicine, however, had sufficient strength to demand that this be done through regional Professional Standards Review Organizations under the complete control of local physicians without even a semblance of patient or community participation in the process. Most of the monitoring remains in the hands of commercial insurance companies or in the hands of the providers themselves, and, not unexpectedly, the wolves have had little success in guarding the sheep.

Meanwhile, national-health-insurance bills proliferated—ranging from a bill sponsored by the AMA which would give tax credits for the voluntary purchase of commercial health insurance; through bills for insurance to cover only catastrophic costs; to a bill introduced by Edward Kennedy and supported by large elements of organized labor, for universal entitlement, comprehensive coverage with few exceptions, little or no out-of-pocket expense at the time of need, significant local control of services, and a period of initial buildup of personnel and facilities to meet the anticipated increased demand for services.

Even the Kennedy proposal, however, fails to address some of the fundamental issues of health protection, of the structure of the medical system, and of equity. While representing a potential improvement over the existing situation and over other proposals, it basically involves pouring even more money into the current system.

Some of the most cogent criticisms of the system during the 1970s have come from the "consumers' movement." The Health Research Group affiliated with Ralph Nader's Public Citizen has produced a series of reports on the dangers and inefficiencies of the U.S. medical-care system, including, for example, criticism of the swine flu immunization program early in its inception. Consumer groups in various cities have produced directories of physicians and hospitals in an attempt to guide patients through the labyrinthine system. Current efforts to rethink ways of dealing with milestones in the life cycle, such as childbirth and dying, which have been largely taken over by technological medicine, are indications of the depth of popular dissatisfaction; and the rapidly growing medical self-help movement represents a clear response to consumer dissatisfaction with the health-care and medical-care system.

Unfortunately, even the most far-reaching of the proposals by the "liberals" would do relatively little to change the basic structure of the system. And the "radical" solutions—including the proposal of a "national health service" for the United States —have as yet gained little public attention.

Social Changes over the Last Quarter-Century and Their Implications for Health Care and Medical Care

Over the last quarter-century U.S. society has been characterized by change so rapid and profound that individuals, families and communities have had considerable difficulty in assimilating and coping with it. The factors that have led to this state of rapid change are manifold, but, while analysts disagree as to their relative importance, there is agreement that the factors are closely interrelated and that together they have had a profound impact on American society and on its need for and provision of health-care and medical-care services.

Urbanization of the United States has been rapid and largely unplanned. According to the U.S. Census Bureau definition, 73 percent of the people in the United States now live in urban areas and only 27 percent in rural areas. This makes the United States one of the world's most urbanized countries; moreover, the growth of metropolitan areas continues, although the patterns of growth are changing. Since 1970 there has been a net internal movement of people from metropolitan areas to non-metropolitan areas, largely to the exurban "fringe," but continued immigration to metropolitan areas from abroad has maintained, although at a slower rate of growth, the long-term trend toward increasing urbanization in the United States.

There has been a marked change, however, in the distribution of people within metropolitan areas. During the 1960s, 15 of the 21 central cities with populations of more than one-half million lost population. During the 1960s and 1970s almost all the growth in metropolitan areas occurred in their suburban areas; currently 13 million more people live in the suburbs than in the cities they surround.

The outmigration of middle- and higher-income families has left the inner cities populated, according to Herbert Gans, by the "cosmopolites," the "unmarried or childless," the "ethnic villagers," the "deprived" and the "trapped and downward mobile." In other terms, the inner-city population predominantly consists of small numbers of the very rich, the poor; working-class ethnic groups; the elderly; and large numbers of blacks and Hispanics. The cities have been left with a severely diminished tax base and an ever-increasing need for services. We have essentially reached the state pictured by President Johnson's Commission on Crimes of Violence:

We can expect further social fragmentation of the urban environment, formation of excessively parochial communities, greater segregation of different racial groups and economic classes . . . and polarization of attitudes on a variety of issues. It is logical to expect the establishment of the "defensive city" consisting of an economically declining central business district in the inner city protected by people shopping or working in buildings during daylight hours and "sealed off" by police during night-time hours. Highrise apartment buildings and residential "compounds" will be fortified "cells" for upper-middle- and high-income populations living at prime locations in the inner city. Suburban neighborhoods, geographically removed from the central city, will be "safe areas," protected mainly by racial and economic homogeneity. . . .

The suburban phenomenon has led to greater discontinuity within families as the younger generation has moved out to the suburbs in search of schools, safety and split-levels, often leaving elderly family members behind in the inner city. At the same time, suburban communities have become, for the most part, enclaves of homogeneity, in which one's neighbors are often at similar stages of the life cycle and are of a similar ethnic and economic group. One observer of contemporary urban America has explained the migration from the cities to the suburbs by stating: "The whole is too large for the individual to comprehend. In the search for self-identity in a mass society, [the individual] seeks to minimize disorder by living in a neighborhood in which life is comprehensible and social relations predictable."

As large numbers of Americans were moving to the suburbs in search of homogeneity and a sense of community, another wave of utopian community-building was taking place. While the first wave of communal experiments was based on a religious critique of society, and the second wave, during the first half of the nineteenth century, was based on a politico-economic critique, the search for new ways of living during the late 1960s and early 1970s was based on a psychosocial critique—that modern society has led to an alienation and isolation of people from society, from one another and even from their own inner feelings. Life in urban America was seen as forcing people to compartmentalize their feelings and to focus on achievement rather than on being or on personal growth. Attempts were therefore made to create communal living situations that would instead foster intimacy, interdependency and a sense of community.

Closely related to the phenomenon of urbanization and suburbanization is the high rate of mobility of a great proportion of the population. As early in the history of the United States as the 1830s Alexis de Tocqueville, in *Democracy in America,* devoted a chapter to "Why the Americans Are Often So Restless in the Midst of Their Prosperity," in which he observed:

> An American will build a house in which to pass his old age and sell it before the roof is on; he will plant a garden and rent it just as the trees are coming into bearing; he will clear a field and leave others to reap the harvest; he will take up a profession and leave it, settle in one place and soon go off elsewhere with his changing desires.

Tocqueville attributed the high rate of geographic mobility to material abundance combined with the lack of a hereditary class structure based on inherited wealth. People in the United States believed, he speculated, that sharing in the abundance was possible through working hard and being willing to move to wherever the opportunities might be found. This trait seemed to Tocqueville to be related to others he found among the American people, including a desire for change, a readiness to accept innovation, and a pragmatic rather than an ideologic basis for action.

Whatever the reason, data for the U.S. census of 1970 indicate that almost 20 percent—one in five—of the people of the United States changed their residence within the previous twelve month period, and about 50 percent had changed their address during the previous five years. The rate of movement was considerably higher than that of Great Britain, with which it was compared in a 1976 Bureau of the Census report; over the year prior to the 1970 census, for example, 11 percent of the British people changed their addresses, compared with 19 percent in the United States. Of the six countries with which the United States was compared, only Australia and Canada had comparably high mobility rates.

Another feature of mobility that emerges from U.S. census data is that if persons have moved once, they are likely to move again. Persons who were living outside their state of birth in 1965, for example, were over three times as likely to move between states in the 1965–70 interval as persons living in their state of birth in 1965.

All in all, the average American has been found to move 14 times during a lifetime, the average Briton 8 times. But the rates differ markedly among social classes; those with higher incomes and greater education who work for large corporate or governmental organizations have a far higher rate of mobility than do working-class people. Alvin Toffler comments in *Future Shock:* "Never have man's relationships with place been more numerous, fragile and temporary. . . . We are witnessing a historic decline in the significance of place to human life. We are breeding a new race of nomads, and few suspect quite how massive, widespread, and significant their migrations are."

At the same time, the size of the American family unit has been steadily shrinking. There are multiple factors at work: Grandparents, aunts and uncles are less likely to live with, or even near, the nuclear family; the large number of divorces and separations produce an increasing number of households each year headed by single parents, frequently women; and the steadily shrinking number of children born to each family. The birth rate in the United States and, more relevant, the fertility rate (the births per year per 1000 women 15–44 years old) has almost halved in 20 years, from about 120 (1 woman in 8 having a baby annually in the 1950s) to 67 (1 in 15) now.

The number of divorces in the United States has risen explosively, from about 100,000 in 1910 to about 200,000 in 1930 to about 400,000 in 1950 to over a million per year now. Stated even more dramatically, the ratio of divorces to marriages has risen from 1:12 in 1910 to 1:6 in 1930 to 1:4 in 1950 to almost 1:2 now. One direct consequence of the fragmented family is the loss of a family network for the promotion of health and for care during illness, and it is often fragmented families who have the greatest medical and social needs.

Another important change is the increasing number and proportion of older people in the population. Those aged 65 and over in the United States have increased from approximately 6 percent of the population 30 years ago to approximately 10 percent of the population now—about 22 million people. The comparative percentages of people aged 65 and over in Sweden and in Britain are 14 percent and 13 percent respectively. It is estimated that by the middle of the next century about 16 percent of the U.S. population—1 in every 6 people—will be 65 or over.

The change in proportion is due in part to the survival of more people in the older age group, but it is mainly due to a decreasing birth rate and therefore fewer numbers of younger people being added to the population. In some areas there are extraordinarily high percentages of older people. The high percentage of people over age 65 in a city like St. Petersburg, Florida, is, of course, due to immigration of older people to the city. In other areas, such as the North Bronx, the extremely high percentage of older people—25 percent of the population in some districts—is due to emigration, the movement of people of working age out of the North Bronx into New Jersey or Westchester, leaving their parents behind. The impact of large numbers of older people, both on social life and on the need and demand for services—particularly medical services—is enormous.

Furthermore, while ours is among the most affluent of the world's societies, there are large numbers of people who do not share in its affluence. In 1976, 10 percent of all families in the United States—25 million people—had incomes below the official "poverty" line even if all income from all public and private sources is included. In 1969, according to the Bureau of the Census, the median income of white families in the United States was $2800 more than black families; in 1974 the difference had increased to $5500 ($13,300 for the white families; $7,800 for the black families). Inadequate housing and nutrition, inadequate education and job opportunities lead to an endless cycle of poverty and illness, of illness and poverty.

In the large cities, particularly, there is also rampant fear. Old people in the North Bronx are literally afraid to step outside their apartments or to open the door to anyone, and for many young people there is also often little feeling of security or safety. Family and community support systems disintegrate and their place is taken by a pervasive feeling of dis-ease.

In this mobile, aging, often socially isolated population, with its extremes of rich and poor, the patterns of disease and death and of the emotional response to them are also changing. At one time the existence of an afterlife was thought to be assured and this life at most a preparation for the next. But in a culture that has become for the most part materialistic and technology-oriented, oriented more to the present or the near future, issues of sickness and health, life and death, have taken on a very different meaning. Ernest Becker has stated that "the idea of death, the fear of it, hunts the human animal like nothing else." He goes on to say that "primitives often celebrate death . . . *because* they believe that death is the ultimate promotion, the final ritual celebration to a higher form of life, to the enjoyment of eternity in some form. Most modern westerners have trouble believing this any more, which is what makes the fear of death so prominent a part of our psychological make-up."

What are the implications for a health-care system of a society whose inhabitants are so fearful of death, who no longer believe death is the "ultimate promotion" to a better form of life? What are the implications for a health-care system of a society for most of whose people health, and medicine, hold out the only hope of "eternal life"?

Along with the fear of death, as Western societies have industrialized, as technology and "progress" and materialism have become more and more a part of our belief system, the technologists have become our new gods. The gods of technology, like the older ones, are thought to be able to "fix" anything and to bring happiness in this life, even if they can't bring salvation in the next. What are the implications for a health-care system of a society most of whose people believe that science and technology can deal with almost anything, given sufficient investment in time and money?

Moreover, some of the new gods are now being found to be false ones. The technological "fix" is found at times to produce more problems than it solves. What are the implications for a health-care system of a society many of whose members view technology—and its attendant institutions—with deepening suspicion and even horror?

The shift from a preponderance of acute infectious disease as the cause of death to a preponderance of chronic, degenerative disease, and the implications of such a shift for health care and medical care, have been discussed in Chapter 1. The prevention of such illness requires community intervention as great or greater than for the prevention of infectious disease; blaming the disease process on individual health habits, and forgetting that these habits are socially and culturally determined, is doomed to failure. Moreover, the care for people with chronic illnesses requires community support far beyond that usually needed for infectious disease; relying on technology and technology-based institutions and personnel to solve what are predominantly problems of social functioning is also doomed to failure. Perhaps not by chance, at the very time that we most need community-based action for health and care, we have it least.

In sum, the current structure of health care and medical care in the United States is, as in other countries, a product of the society's history and of its political, social, economic and cultural structure. But, as we saw in Chapter 1, medical care in the United States has grown increasingly dysfunctional and incapable of meeting the changing needs brought about by changes in societal patterns and illness patterns. In the final chapter we attempt to formulate some recommendations which may permit it to begin to do so, and to be a leading edge in other social change as well.

7

PROPOSALS AND PROSPECTS

As we discussed in our introduction, it is our view that the purposes of a society's health-care and medical-care system go beyond the conventional definitions of protection of people's health and care for those who are ill. We have summarized these purposes in four areas:

1. an increase in equity and justice
2. a strengthening of individual, family and community competence and well-being
3. the protection and promotion of health
4. the organization and provision of humane and technologically appropriate care for the sick and the "worried well"

Before we explore the ways in which the U.S. health-care and medical-care system can be changed, it is important to state yet again that the formal health-care and medical-care system is only one, and not the most important one, of society's methods for approaching these four goals, including the last two. Redistribution of power and income are far more important, obviously in relation to the first goals, but also in relation to health and to care. Nonetheless we believe that the health-care and medical-care system can contribute significantly toward reaching all of these goals or, conversely, can be an impediment to reaching them.

It appears to us that the health-care and medical-care systems of the other countries we have described, despite the continuing problems they face, attempt to reach these goals, and succeed in doing so, to a far greater extent than does the health-care and medical-care system of the United States. In this final chapter we wish to explore some of the ways in which our system might be restructured so as to contribute more fully to these goals.

While techniques for providing health care and medical care surely cannot be transplanted from one society to another, a number of fundamental principles have emerged from our examination of the systems in Sweden, Great Britain, the Soviet Union and China which we feel are essential to any restructuring of the system in the United States. Sweden's attempts at regionalization and its efforts in preventive medicine; Great Britain's commitment to equity in provision of care and to the maintenance of community-based primary care; the Soviet Union's guarantee of basic health care and medical care to its entire population without charge at the time of service and with special attention to target populations; and China's extensive use of paraprofessional health workers and community workers to provide health care and medical care—all are examples of ways in which health care and medical care can further the goals we consider urgent within each society's total framework.

In this final part of the book we will present a set of principles for the future of health care and medical care in the United States which we believe incorporates the relevant aspects of the experience of other countries and structures them in the context of our own society and its experience. We are already—as we shall show—closer to an equitable, caring, workable system in the United States than those who oppose it would have us believe. On the other hand, since it is unlikely that the entire system can be put into place in the near future, we will offer a number of recommendations for short-run change which will lead us toward—rather than away from—an appropriate total system of health care and medical care.

Long-term Goals

Overall, nothing short of a national health service can help us to approach the goals we seek in a consistent and meaningful way. Since funding by insurance premiums or even flat-rate social security payments tends to take funds inequitably from the poor, a national health service must be funded by "progressive taxation," so that the *source* of the funds serves to help redistribute wealth.

The *expenditures* in the service must also help to redistribute wealth. Profit-making in the health-care and medical-care system appears to us particularly incompatible with the goal of equity and is incompatible with the goals of community, health, and humane care as well. Two of the four countries we have discussed have systems with few if any profit-making elements in the economy, and the other two have sharply limited or regulated profit-making in health care. We reject it as a basis for the organization of any part of health care or medical care in the United States; a national health service must not permit investors to gain wealth or income at the expense of the sick or at the expense of the rest of the society. This of course extends to insurance companies and drug companies as well as to profit-making entrepreneurs in hospitals, nursing homes and ambulatory care.

Since accountability to the community and to the society at large is critical in its performance, the service must be under direct public control. It must have nationally set policies and standards, with effective mechanisms to see that they are met, for only in this way can resources appropriately be distributed to help increase equity on a national scale and can national priorities for community development, health and care be set. But much decision-making on local priorities, all of the implementation, and much of the evaluation of how well the program is meeting the needs set for it must be performed locally. This local control has two purposes. On the one hand, it makes the health-care system more responsive to local needs and reduces bureaucratic entanglements; on the other hand, and even more important, it fosters community competence and cohesion in solving community problems.

Because fee-for-service medicine spawns sporadic, individual, technical services, it is largely incompatible with long-term supportive care for chronic illness and is also incompatible with planned preventive medicine, which must work with the community as a whole rather than simply with those who request care. Since, as we have seen, so much of current illness in the United States is induced by environmental and social factors and so much of it is chronic in nature, the fee-for-service model of organizing medical care, if it ever had any validity, is increasingly anachronistic. And, of course, fee-for-service medicine is one of the prime causes of the abuses of the system—abuses such as the overuse of surgery and other medical services and the corruption of both physicians and patients in seeking reimbursement.

One or more of the prepaid alternatives to fee-for-service, such as capitation payments (as for the GP in Great Britain) or salaries (as for consultants in Britain, most health workers in Sweden and all health workers in China and the USSR), must be used as the method of compensation for services rendered. But building on the pluralism which has characterized the history of our medical-care system, there is every reason, within the prepayment framework, to "let a hundred flowers bloom." Many different forms of reimbursement can be accommodated, and evaluated to determine their impact on patient care, on efficiency and cost and on physician satisfaction.

The focus for a national health service must be the community health center rather than either the hospital, the individual doctor's office or the health department. This model, advocated in Britain as early as the 1920s, institutionalized in the USSR in the 1930s and given a new meaning in China since 1950, was explored in the United States—for the poor—through the Office of Economic Opportunity and Department of Health,

Education and Welfare health centers of the 1960s. In a national health service, primary medical care should be given through neighborhood centers which also house integrated health, social and welfare services. Furthermore, strong links must be built between the community health centers and other social institutions such as schools, places of work and community organizations.

The goal is not to "medicalize" these groups, but rather to enable them to contribute more fully to the health of their members and to enable them to play a role in the shaping of the community health system. The community health center must be a part of the community, must be a facilitating institution which enables people to deal with their health needs more effectively. Its focus must not be primarily technical—although appropriate technical skills must be available when they are needed—but communal, social and environmental. Again, many different models can be accommodated, from the individual physician working in a small isolated town with one or two other health or social-welfare workers, to a group of primary-care physicians practicing together in a densely crowded urban area with many different types of social and health services integrated into the practice.

A *sine qua non* of an effective community health center is a defined community in which health work is to be done. The health workers in the center must be responsible for overseeing the health care and medical care of all of the people in the community. Strong referral links to specified secondary- and tertiary-care institutions for consultation and referral must be present. This does not mean that individuals in the community cannot seek primary or more specialized care from other sources if they wish. It does mean, however, that there should be no additional cost to the public if they do so.

One or two patients moving outside the geographic boundaries to another primary-care site because of "incompatibility" between patient and doctor or other health workers can be accommodated; large numbers of patients doing so means that something in the primary-care system is amiss and must be altered. And even one or two patients deciding that they want to go to a hospital which does not serve the geographic referral area may be too many if expensive services are sought.

Indeed technological medical care has become so expensive and hazardous that free choice for quality care may have to give way to a structured and defined system. This will mean that patients and referring doctors will not have access, as now, to any cardiac surgeon who will accept the patient; instead communities and primary-care doctors will have to make certain that the specialists who serve the area are technically competent and humane, and will have to retrain them or replace them if they are not.

Those practicing medical care should whenever possible be organized into groups or teams so that health care and medical care can be effectively integrated and so that health workers' skills can be used as effectively and efficiently as possible. Again, many different models for such teams can be accommodated and evaluated. Real teamwork, however, is only feasible if the physician takes his or her place as one health worker among many, with a particular and valuable set of skills, to be sure, but without the dominant role that the physician now plays. In order to facilitate a more egalitarian relationship among health workers—as well as to reduce the social distance between physicians and most of their patients—the goal must be to bring physicians' incomes more in line with the income of other health workers, or at least to freeze them until the incomes of others rise significantly.

The hospital should be reserved for use as a technical institution for diagnosis and treatment of medical problems that cannot be handled in other ways. This is true not only because of the high cost to society of operating hospitals but also because of the human cost of high technology and of institutionalization. Hospitals, or in some instances parts of the same hospital, must be separated into "secondary care" institutions, tied closely to the community, for diagnosis and treatment requiring relatively less complex equipment and training, and "tertiary care" institutions in which the most complex technological equipment and personnel are regionalized for those patients who truly need that level of care.

The hospital system in short, must be rationalized to meet patient needs and not, as now, to augment the prestige, and often the incomes, of the professionals. This of course means eliminating all profit-making in hospitals, and probably even more important it means that all hospitals must be regionalized and brought under effective public ownership and control. As in the health centers, health workers must be reeducated and organized to work together in less hierarchical ways for the benefit of the hospitalized patient and for effective communication with patients, with families and with the community physician and other health workers who will work with the patient after discharge from the hospital.

At all levels of the system, appropriate technology and appropriate use of it should be assured. This means that some of the incentives to overuse of technology—such as profit, or fear of malpractice suits—must be eliminated from the system.

To work in this new kind of system both outside and inside the hospital, a new breed of health worker will be needed. For equity as well as effectiveness in communication with patients for health and care, they must be more representative of the community they will serve. For strengthening of the community, they must be trained in ways that emphasize community activity and sharing of responsibility for care, rather than either technology or custodial care, both of them dependency-producing.

To meet these goals physicians must be chosen in far greater numbers from among the poor or the working class, from among females, blacks and other relatively disadvantaged groups, from among people who relate to others in caring, egalitarian modes, rather than in technical, dominant modes. Their training must emphasize their accessibility to the community and to other health workers, rather than merely to other doctors and to their individual patients. Their training must also provide skills that permit them to work effectively in teams, subordinating their own views and needs, to those of others when necessary. That this can be done in a shorter period of time than is considered necessary by most schools in the United States has been demonstrated in the countries we have studied as well as in a number of schools here.

Moreover, this education must be provided at no cost to the student—and with appropriate stipends during training—if we are to recruit students from new pools and if we are to avoid a vicious cycle of high personal costs of education followed by demands for ever higher income. Furthermore the privilege of obtaining this education incurs the obligation of serving, at least for a defined period of time, where the needs are greatest.

But it is not enough to change the selection and training patterns of physicians; the selection and training patterns of other health workers must also be fundamentally changed. While those who were formerly dominant must be selected, trained and rewarded in ways that make them less dominant, those whose roles have been traditionally subservient must be recruited, trained and rewarded for playing less subservient roles. Males, blacks and members of other minority groups must be recruited into nursing, and nurses must be trained to be more confident, assertive, willing to see themselves as partners in providing care. The recruitment, training, and working conditions of other types of health workers who are now poorly paid and poorly regarded must be changed so that they are able to function as significant, respected members of the health team.

Communities must play a far more significant role in the decision-making and in the evaluation of health services. This will require a much higher level of knowledge of—and willingness to take continuing responsibility for—technical, financial, administrative and medical-care issues.

Individual patients, too, must take a far higher level of responsibility for their own care. The patient must participate in the decisions which are now largely being made by physicians or other health workers about his or her care, and the participation must be based on sharing and demystifying all the information relevant to the decision. One of the ways of fostering this in a national health service is to give each patient a standardized copy of his or her own medical record, as is frequently done in China. This is an especially valuable technique in a society with high mobility, and also facilitates exchange of information between those providing primary care and those providing secondary or tertiary care.

A national health service must itself provide, or be closely linked to the agencies which provide, environmental protection and health education. Far higher priority, and therefore a far higher level of funding, must be given to primary prevention and the measures used must be tied as closely as possible to community, family, and individual action on the one hand and, through the community health centers, to the medical-care system on the other.

Occupational health and safety must also be given major new importance. Again, workers in their individual workplaces must have increased responsibilities for their own health, within appropriate national guidelines and with education in the technical and administrative aspects of occupational health. Health-care and medical-care services in work settings must be a formal part of a national health service and must have strong ties to the community health centers where the worker's family —and at times the worker himself or herself—receives care.

Lest this outline of a national health service for the United States seem utopian and unachievable, we must state our conviction that it is inevitable and entirely consistent with our historic development, although those who currently control resources and power in American medicine clearly will not relinquish them without a struggle. While we as a nation have often betrayed our dream, we feel that the United States has had from its beginings the dream of "justice for all." Even if it is kept alive for long periods of time only by rhetoric and mythology, the belief in a more equitable distribution of the riches of this land has been a consistent part of our national ideology.

Furthermore, constructing a national health service, with national funding, national allocation of resources and national setting of guidelines in order to increase justice and equity, is well within the framework of the American experience—particularly if much of the implementation is left under local control. For while centralized control has often been viewed with suspicion within American society, centralized standard setting tempered by local administration and varied implementation relevant to local needs, is workable, we believe, within the American context.

The same can be said even more strongly for a search for and belief in community. Much of the past 200 years can be characterized as a search for a mode of living in which citizens with similar values and ideology could live together and build a congenial environment. From the first settlers with their covenants through which they spelled out their ideal society; to the utopians who withdrew from society to build their own communities; to the waves of immigrants who, upon settling in the New World, formed homogeneous enclaves partly out of necessity, partly out of choice; to the post–World War II urban exodus to the suburbs—Americans have been seeking a way of living together and building workable institutions. While the search for community in America has often been a rural dream, ways must be found to translate that dream into an urban reality.

A thread of antielitism has run parallel in the United States to the belief in the natural superiority of the elite. The antielitist strain in medicine enabled a great variety of health workers to function beside "regular" doctors until late in the nineteenth century. This willingness to view health care and medical care as the province of the many rather than the task of the few has also been evident in the important role voluntary organizations have played in the health field and has led to the recent attempts to develop new kinds of health workers and to find ways for people to help themselves and one another through the self-help movement.

Finally, a strain of optimism permeates American history—the belief that all is possible, that all is conquerable (a belief which in perverted forms can cause tragedies such as the Vietnam War). This belief has been transferred to a profound faith in the efficacy of technology. While severe problems stem from our worship of the technological "fix," the widespread view that all should benefit from the riches of American technology can be utilized in building a health-care and medical-care system that is both technologically appropriate and just.

Moreover, despite some of the myths about our present system, it is closer in many ways to the one we seek than those who have vested interests in keeping it from changing would have us believe. It is widely believed, for example, that medicine is an entrepreneurial, self-employed, "small business" profession, yet it is estimated that one-fourth or more of all doctors in the United States already work on a salaried basis, and the percentage grows annually.

It is also widely believed that medical care is purchased by individuals from the physician or institution of their choice, yet 40 percent of the funding for health care and medical care comes from tax funds and an additional 30 percent comes from communal, pooled insurance funds. Indeed, large groups of the population are already directly served by a public medical-care system, such as by Veterans Administration or armed forces medical care or by municipal and county hospital systems.

It is widely believed that medicine is predominantly a male profession, yet today 15 percent of all U.S. doctors are women, and 25 percent of incoming medical-school classes are female.

It is widely believed that doctors are free to practice wherever they wish, yet the increasingly large numbers of doctors whose education is paid for by government agencies such as the armed forces or the National Health Service Corps give up a considerable degree of autonomy on where and how they will practice for at least part of their careers.

It is widely believed that doctors pay for their own medical education and should therefore be free to earn as much as the traffic will bear, yet over half of the costs of medical education are already borne by government at one level or another or indirectly by payments for patient care, and for some students almost all expenses are already covered by one government agency or another.

Furthermore, recent changes, or contemplated changes, in health care and medical care have the potential to bring us closer to a national health-care and medical-care system that will meet our goals. The National Health Planning and Resources Development Act of 1974 is bringing each region of the United States a Health Systems Agency which at least in theory gives communities the power to shape some elements of the system through the local allocation of federal funds. The National Health Service Corps will markedly expand the number of physicians it places in "medically underserved areas." National health insurance, which began with Medicare and Medicaid, is also on the way to significant expansion.

These changes, and others that will be taking place to meet every newly found defect in a part of the system, can be a force for good or ill depending on the way they affect the health-care and medical-care system as a whole. Health Systems Agencies can be simply a facade for control of the system by those who now control it and by their technicians, or they can truly explore new forms of community participation in health-care planning. The National Health Service Corps can be simply a patching operation to cover some of the worst holes in the system, thereby delaying significant change, or it can provide models and can be a step toward real change. National health insurance—and new categorical programs for care—can be steps toward or away from our goals depending on whether they begin to reshape the system or simply further ossify it or increase the inequities that we currently have.

Short-term Goals

What are some of the steps we can take now or in the next year or so—steps that are politically, socially, culturally and economically feasible—that will bring us closer to our goal? And as we take these steps, how can we avoid further fragmentation of the system and further inequity?

1. *Promotion and Protection of Health*

Movement toward the promotion of health and the prevention of illness can be made in ways that themselves promote equity and community and lead toward a national health service that further promotes these goals. Examples may be found in a number of different areas.

Environmental protection. Some environmental pollutants are now well known to cause cancer of the respiratory system, the liver and the bladder or other illnesses. For other substances, where the toxic hazard is not yet proven, there are reasonable grounds for suspicion. In either of these circumstances there is often insufficient information to determine what level of exposure, if any, is "safe." Appropriate research on toxicity must be done, with far greater priority than it is now accorded. In the meantime, when there is dispute or doubt, every effort should be made to protect the public against known or suspected hazards.

This, of course, often generates conflict with those who benefit from the process that leads to the hazard, either as investors, managers, consumers or, most difficult of all, workers in the industry that produces the hazard. The conflict can be resolved in favor of health by strong enough pressure from groups of people concerned with protection of the environment who act in concert with each other—an expression of community. Ways must be developed to provide other, less environmentally destructive methods of earning income for workers. As Barry Commoner and others have pointed out, there is no fundamental conflict between full employment and environmental protection if production for social usefulness rather than for profit is the controlling element. In the meantime, more effective controls on production processes that produce pollutants and controls on products that are unnecessarily environmentally destructive can begin to move us in the right direction.

If these efforts were also coordinated with an effort to build a national health service—by demonstrating how the current health-care and medical-care system is incapable of dealing effectively with such issues and that current proposals for change in the health-care system fall far short of being able to deal with them—both the efforts for environmental protection and the efforts to change the health-care and medical-care system could be strengthened.

Occupational health and safety. There is little doubt that only the workers themselves, acting initially in their own self-interest and then in the interest of others, can effectively protect their own health and safety. Yet most activity in occupational health involves attempts at regulation and control from outside the factory rather than attempts to give the workers themselves the knowledge and the skills to study the hazards and to devise production changes or protective methods which will reduce the hazard. In fact in many factories the nature of the chemicals the workers deal with is an "industrial secret" that is kept even from them. The absence of an effective industrial health-care and medical-care system, or else its control by management, prevents workers from learning about the numbers and types of illnesses being uncovered among fellow workers.

The development of health and medical services in the industrial sector can provide models for the organization of care for a defined population and for maximizing the participation of that population in the planning, provision and evaluation of their own care. Furthermore, occupational health- and medical-care services can be designed for later integration into a national health service rather than further fragmenting the current system or acting as a barrier to the implementation of a comprehensive one.

Health education. Since a considerable amount of responsibility for the protection of health and prevention of illness lies in the hands of the individual, strong efforts must be instituted in this area. There is little evidence that current formal methods of health education are effective in changing habits and practices from those known to be destructive to health to those which will promote it. Some of the most successful efforts lie outside the formal education system and are conducted by community groups and in peer networks. These health-education efforts at the community level can be encouraged and strengthened, thus promoting community cohesion and laying the groundwork for expanded community participation in health care and medical care. At the same time, centralized services can be developed for support of local efforts through information-gathering on risks, methods of education, production of teaching materials, and comparative evaluation of the success of various efforts.

But it is not enough for society with one hand to try to undo damage which, with the other hand, it permits certain interests in the society to continue to cause. Cigarette smoking is a classic example. So long as tobacco companies are permitted through advertising to seduce people into starting—and continuing—to smoke, little good will be done by "education" against smoking. Local communities are usually powerless to stop the flood of printed, billboard and other material which attempts to link smoking with the vigorous outdoor life, sex and other pleasures. This merchandising of death and disability must be stopped centrally—as in the ban on cigarette advertising on television.

Immunization. The shamefully low level of immunization against preventable communicable disease in the United States can be used as a vehicle to move toward a true community health system that involves every individual in the community. The clear failure of the current health- and medical-care system to provide adequate levels of immunization, and the clear increase in inequity caused by current methods of distribution, provide opportunities for community organization of immunization efforts through local organizations, residential networks and school systems. These efforts must be designed to reach every member of the community and, again, can serve, as we have seen in China, as organizing tools both for community cohesion and for the development of community participation in an effective health- and medical-care system.

Clearly the education of community members, the medical and administrative elements needed for such an immunization program, and appropriate supervision must be provided by the health-care system. Merely placing the responsibility for such programs on local communities without the necessary planning, equipment and backup—free of charge—serves ultimately to increase inequity rather than to promote equity.

Screening for asymptomatic illness. For a few illnesses, though not as many as the medical profession would like us to believe, there is evidence that early detection and appropriate treatment can lead to prevention of symptoms or complications, or at least to delay in their progression. Examples of illnesses which current evidence suggests can be modified by early detection are hypertension, glaucoma and—although the evidence is less clear—certain cancers, such as those of the breast and of the uterus. In addition, for some illnesses—such as tuberculosis and venereal disease—danger to others as well as to the individual affected can be prevented.

For these kinds of illnesses efforts can be mounted—through community organizations and through individual physicians and medical institutions—to provide appropriate screening. But the screening will only be effective in the immediate protection of health and in building toward an effective system if appropriate linkages for follow-up and treatment are provided for those found to need it. This is an example of an important interface between health care and medical care, one at which much less is being done to provide integration than would be possible even within our current fragmented system.

In short, all of these efforts—in environmental protection, occupational health and safety, health education, immunization, screening and others—should be made in ways that lead us toward an integrated system of health care and medical care rather than away from it. This integration is conceptually and practically far less simple than it might superficially seem. For example, what is the medical-care system's—and the physician's—responsibility with regard to the child who has been bitten by a rat in the tenement in which his family lives?

One view holds that the child who comes to a physician or a hospital with rat bite at that point becomes the full health-care and medical-care responsibility of the physician or institution, and the responsibility does not end when the rat bite has been properly sutured. This school of thought says that the agents of the medical-care system have responsibilities for health care as well, that they have responsibility for doing something about the rats, that it is "bad medicine" to send the child back to the same tenement in which he, and his brothers and sisters, will be bitten by rats.

The opposition to this view says that taking care of the rats —or the lead paint on the walls or the fire hazards—is a function best left to elements outside of the "medical-care system," that physicians and medical-care institutions have little knowledge or skill in dealing with rats or landlords or vermin exterminators, and that at most the physician's responsibility extends to making the environmental hazard known to those whose professional or social responsibility it is to deal with it.

Another example of the dispute about the role of "medical care" lies in the extent to which the physician or other "medical" worker should have the power to enforce—or even to strongly urge—healthful behavior on the part of the patient or the family. H. L. Mencken stated the dichotomy pungently:

> Hygiene is the corruption of medicine by morality. It is impossible to find a hygienist who does not debase his theory of the healthful with a theory of the virtuous. The whole hygienic art, indeed, resolves itself into an ethical exhortation. This brings it, at the end, into diametrical conflict with medicine proper. The true aim of medicine is not to make men virtuous; it is to safeguard and rescue them from the consequences of their vices. The physician does not preach repentence; he offers absolution.

Concern about these inherent tensions between the health-care and medical-care roles should not be ignored. Although there are considerable areas of overlap, medical care is largely concerned with helping those who come to the system for help; health care is concerned with protecting the health of the entire community. Medical care is concerned largely with the individual, trying to maximize the individual patient's well-being and, when necessary, mobilizing additional social resources for his or her particular benefit; health care is concerned largely with the community, trying to maximize the well-being of all the individuals within it. Medicine is concerned largely with trying to undo what is done; health with trying to keep it from happening.

Appealing in some ways as this dichotomous analysis may be, it is an analysis with serious flaws. If Mencken's "vices" lead to illnesses whose treatment and other consequences cost everyone else in the society billions of dollars, they are unquestionably of deep concern to the entire society and to its medical-care system. As medical care increasingly comes to be viewed as a "right" rather than as a privilege to be bought and paid for, and as broadly based social insurance or taxation bears more of the cost, the responsibility for maintaining one's personal health becomes more "social" than "individual" and the dividing line between health care and sick care becomes even hazier.

There is also a practical point: The occasion of sick care can often be a critical moment in the life of the patient. It can be a moment at which the patient is ready to listen to advice about change of habits or life-style, or even about the ways in which inequity, social fragmentation, environmental hazards and other social problems have led to the illness. Medicine can be a wedge for changes in the individual and in the society which can bring us closer to health.

Again we are brought back to the fundamental question of the structure of the system. Attempts to resolve these problems piecemeal, without a vision of a system in which health care and medical care are integrated and community-based rather than individual-patient-based, are doomed to failure. In a community-ty-based system there can be appropriate division of responsibility among the various groups concerned with health—the members of the medical team; nonmedical specialists such as the environmentalist, the health educator, the lawyer and the vermin exterminator; and community residents, activists and nonprofessional health workers. The sharing of the responsibility for health with all sectors of the community will not only serve the goal of promotion and protection of health but will help to deprofessionalize and demystify medicine and can serve as a tool for advancing equity and a stronger sense of community.

2. *Organization of Medical Care*

Just as there are many different ways in which short-term efforts in health care, short of a national health service, can—if the overall goals are kept clearly in view—lead toward the broader goals we seek, there are short-term efforts in medical care which can lead in appropriate directions if their ultimate purpose is clear.

Development of prepaid group practice. It has been repeatedly shown that prepaid group practices like Kaiser-Permanente hospitalize their members far less often, do much less surgery and practice considerably more preventive medicine than do most physicians who are paid by fee-for-service or who are not in group practice. The cost saving which this pattern of care produces was the basis of the encouragement of Health Maintenance Organizations (HMOs) by the Nixon administration, but one of the features, not surprisingly, of the current regulations of HMOs is that there can be profit-making and that they need take no responsibility for low-income neighborhoods which cannot sustain the costs. If these defects were removed, the prepaid, community-based group practice, particularly if tied to a neighborhood health center, might be a viable model for the provision of health services under a national health service.

Prepaid group practice—with hospitals as integral parts of the system so that the savings on hospitalization can be shifted into ambulatory care—is only one of the ways in which ambulatory care can be fostered and hospitalization reduced. Expansion of insurance coverage and benefits for ambulatory care, for example, will reduce hospitalization for procedures that are presently only covered by insurance if performed in the hospital.

One of the methods which will *not* lead in the appropriate direction, however, is the arbitrary setting of ceilings on costs or the reduction of services in the name of "keeping costs down." Such reductions will always hurt those patients who have the least. The wealthy and the powerful can usually find ways to gain access to scarce resources; the poor will invariably be the ones shunted aside. Under a national health service it would be possible to reduce the number of hospital beds and other costly services because firm control of regionalization and referral will assure that the remaining services are equitably utilized. In the absence of such a system, care must be taken that reductions in some services follow rather than precede the provision of more appropriate services, and thus promote equity and protect the needs of communities rather than undermine them.

Changes in hierarchies within institutions. Great difficulties impede the modification of the hierarchical structure of medical-care institutions. The enormous wage and status differentials between physicians and other health workers, the financing and service structures of the institutions, licensure restrictions and fear of malpractice suits, and the models from other institutions in the society all make the patterns difficult to break.

Nonetheless, in some medical-care settings, particularly in the neighborhood health centers funded by the federal government in the 1960s, attempts were made to introduce and strengthen team practice of medicine and to encourage new roles and relationships. Within the constraints that the broader society and the structure of individual institutions impose, efforts in this direction may in the short run lead to a diminution of "efficiency." So long as the ultimate goals are served, such short-term problems can be tolerated or even welcomed as a part of the process of change.

Fostering "appropriate" use of technology. Control must be increasingly imposed over the technological elements of the system, both to curb runaway costs and to keep patients from harm. Each element of technology will require its own pattern of controls. Diagnostic techniques, such as specific types of X-ray and laboratory tests, and cardiac catheterization, exploratory surgery and other invasive methods will have to be limited in their use to the level of the system at which they are needed and at which there is adequate competence in their use.

The problem is even more critical in the area of treatment techniques. Controls on surgeons—through "second opinions," limitation of surgical privileges to those with adequate training and skill, and insistence that an adequate amount of each type of surgery be performed to maintain skills—are urgently needed and will move the system toward stronger and more effective controls. The most widespread problem, however, is that of the cost and adverse consequences of the use of drugs, both by prescription and over the counter. A variety of methods are available to attempt to deal with the problem. These include: using standardized lists of drugs and prescribing by generic rather than brand name to establish competence in the use of a limited number of drugs and to reduce the unnecessary costs of producing and stocking redundant drugs; restricting advertising and other forms of drug promotion by drug companies, again both for protection of the patient and for cost control; establishment of a strict reporting system for efficacy of drugs and adverse drug reactions; and education of the population on the appropriate indications and the contraindications for use of specific drugs and on the appropriate questions to ask before using drugs.

A large part of the control must lie in regionalization of scarce and expensive services. In our society, in which relatively few general hospitals are now operated by government, only a national health service will be able to provide true regionalization along the lines used in all the countries we have studied—including Sweden, where almost all the hospitals are government-owned. Nonetheless, even in our current system some steps can be taken through the use of the mechanism provided by government and insurance funding. As we have discussed however, arbitrary closing or restriction of services without attention to equity or community patterns of care in the use of those that are left, while perhaps "cost-saving" in the short run, will almost certainly move the system away from the long-term goals.

The other side of the coin of "appropriate" technology are those methods felt to be efficacious by some people but rejected on the basis of "lack of scientific merit" by most physicians. The problem has been approached in China, as we have seen, by cross-training doctors of "Western" medicine in "Chinese" medicine and doctors of "Chinese" medicine in "Western" medicine. This solution has the advantage of making available to the patient those elements of either system which might be of help. Where such a combination does not exist, there is danger that the patient may be deprived of a symptom-relieving or even life-saving method from either the "regular" or the "alternative" system.

In a national health service such combinations can be formally built into the system, but in the meantime patients who use one or the other must be protected by full disclosure of information on available alternatives. The patient, for example, who gets no relief from muscle or joint pain from the "regular" system must be told that acupuncture or other forms of alternative treatment have helped other patients with that same condition. Conversely, ways must be found, even in the short run, to insure that the patient who is using the alternative system is aware that the regular system may have forms of effective treatment available.

Collection of data needed for planning. An important step that can be taken now to form the foundation for planning an effective national health service is the collection of data on medical-care needs and on the utilization and outcome of various elements in the medical-care system. As a requirement of the licensure of medical-care practitioners and medical-care institutions there must be regular and consistent supplying of information on the nature of the problems for which patients are seeking care and on the treatment given and its results. Computer technology now exists that is capable of storing and analyzing such masses of data.

Even these efforts, which would appear to be among the least controversial of our recommendations, will be resisted on several grounds. Many will argue, for example, that the collection of such data will interfere with the "autonomy" of the professional. This argument is easily refuted: Not only is it not clear that professionals should have as much uncontrolled latitude to diagnose and treat as they now have, but it is not clear how the simple collection of data interferes with their autonomy. The argument is usually a cover for another, less socially acceptable reason for resistance to revealing such data: fear of exposure of incompetence, or of income on which taxes have not been paid.

The more difficult argument to counter is that of the danger of disclosure of information which the patient wishes kept confidential. One way to protect patients would be to make certain that no information is collected that specifically identifies the patient. This protection will work for the collection of some data and is certainly a good starting point, but really effective use of the information would involve linking the data supplied by, for example, the primary-care physician on a patient with cancer with the data supplied on the same patient by a radiotherapy or a surgical unit. The linking of the data requires identification of the individual patient, and even if done by number rather than by name, raises the possibility of unauthorized disclosure rather than use simply for statistical planning and evaluation. Furthermore, a linked set of records often contains much more information about an individual than the records of any one of the practitioners or institutions supplying the data, and disclosure may therefore be more harmful. It will thus be necessary to move cautiously when dealing with identified and linked data. But this caution should not stand in the way of immediate efforts to collect data not tied identifiably to specific individuals while developing more secure methods for safeguarding data on individuals.

One more point should be made about data collection. It is no accident, as we pointed out in Chapter 1, that very few data are available on the differences in health status and the use of health-care and medical-care services by social class. Another step toward our goals would be to insist that data on, for example, infant and maternal mortality, age-specific death rates, morbidity rates, disability rates and rates of use of health services be collected not on the basis of "race"—which often is difficult to define and the use of which may lead to misinterpretation and negative consequences—but on the basis of "class." There is now a sufficient base of sociological and economic thought for appropriate definitions of "class" to be formulated and used in a standardized way. The impact of collecting the data in this way may be as powerful as the efforts of Griscom in New York City and Shattuck in Boston a century ago in making clear some of the causes of poor health and of inequities in distribution of services.

3. *National Health Insurance*

Since implementation of some form of national health insurance appears likely in the near future, it is important to analyze its likely impact on movement toward our goals.

A number of the current proposals will clearly move us in the wrong direction: These include proposals that emphasize medical care at the expense of preventive medicine, and hospital care at the expense of ambulatory care, such as the proposals for "catastrophic-illness insurance."

Another group of proposals would leave the current practice of medicine essentially unmodified and uncontrolled or leave unchanged the role of the insurance companies; these, of course, are offered respectively by the AMA and by the insurance industry. These proposals, and others, impose significant deductible and coinsurance payments on patients and families at the time of illness in the name of "keeping down costs," a code phrase for rationing care—more bluntly, for keeping people from getting the care they think they need—through the use of financial barriers rather than education on appropriate use. Financial barriers, of course, diminish equity and community as well as, through their irrationality, health and care.

There is only one plan that has wide support—from organized labor, from groups of older citizens, from the "liberal" establishment in medicine—and seems designed in any significant way to avoid these problems and to approach our goals. It is the Health Security bill, introduced as the Kennedy-Griffiths bill in 1971 and now called, in somewhat revised form, the Kennedy-Corman bill. This bill would eliminate the role of insurance companies, would eliminate deductible and coinsurance payments, would encourage regionalization and more equitable distribution of large segments of medicine, would encourage group practice, would provide an entry point for public representation in the area of quality of care and in allocation of funding, and would use a largely "progressive" system of taxation as its source of funds.

However, this proposal is also flawed in a number of ways: There are limitations on coverage of psychiatric care, dental care, skilled nursing-home care, and drugs; the possibilities are limited for shifting resources from one area to another or for adding resources in areas of greatest need; and it cannot deal with some of the glaring structural defects in the system. Most important, since its control of the system is largely through financing rather than operation, it carries the danger of further inflation of medical-care costs and the danger of use of the services in ways which continue to serve the interests of the professionals or of the institutions.

Another type of approach, suggested by some of the advisers to the Carter administration, is related to legislation proposed by Congressman Scheuer and Senator Javits. They urge concentration on one area—maternal and child care—as a "first phase" in national health insurance. While a Carter program has not yet been formulated at the time of this writing, it seems likely that it will be more limited than Kennedy-Corman both in the range of its coverage and in its ability to bring needed structural change into even this limited part of the system.

Finally, a number of small groups have in recent years been going beyond advocacy of national health insurance to advocacy of a national health service. These groups include, for example, a "liberal" physicians' group (Physicians Forum), a more "radical" group of physicians and other health workers (Medical Committee for Human Rights), a policy-study group (the Community Health Alternatives Project of the Institute for Policy Studies) and a committee composed of health workers and others specifically organized to work toward a national health service (Committee for a National Health Service). These efforts have been hindered by internal disputes and by difficulties in finding congressional sponsors, although Congressman Ronald Dellums has been supportive of some of the efforts and has introduced a bill embodying some principles of a national health service.

Even among those who think that a national health service is the only way to solve the United States' health-care and medical-care problems, an argument rages about the best way to achieve it. Some critics, from both the political right and left, argue that the idea of a national health service is too "utopian" to be either educationally or politically useful, and that advocating it will simply lead to "frustration." The advocates argue that the concept is useful educationally, as a method of clarifying the flaws in the various national health-insurance plans, and that it is useful politically, as a rallying point for those who feel that national health insurance will not itself solve the problems and may aggravate them. An important step toward credibility for the proposal was a statement in October 1976 by four past presidents of the American Public Health Association:

> We are fearful that a national health insurance measure will be enacted into law which will repeat the serious mistakes of Medicare and Medicaid, and which will fail to address the really critical issues confronting this nation with respect to health care for the people. All of the many proposals introduced in Congress which are described as national health insurance bills are essentially financial mechanisms for providing guaranteed payments to the providers of health care services, and they contain virtually no provisions for the reform or alteration of the American health care system. It has become more and more apparent, not only to health professionals and scholars but to much of the general public, that there are fundamental flaws in our system of providing health services which must not be incorporated into a new health system.

Our own position is that it is not inconsistent to work for the Kennedy-Corman bill, as the most comprehensive of the politically "possible" national health-insurance plans and one with wide support in the community, and, at the same time, as we are doing in this book, to advocate a national health service as the only rational long-term solution to our problems.

4. *Control of the "Quality of Medical Care"*

Present methods for measurement and control of quality of medical care put almost all of the power in this area into the hands of medical professionals through Professional Standards Review Organizations or "peer review" audit committees. Not only does this mean that the definitions of quality, and therefore the methods chosen, will be oriented toward the perceptions and the goals of the professionals, but it also means that the methods in large measure will be chosen on the basis of criteria with which technically trained professionals are comfortable—

methods with a high degree of precision, reliability and reproducibility.

Since some characteristics of care are relatively easy to measure, usually from the patient's record—for example, whether an electrocardiogram (ECG) was taken for a patient with chest pain, how well the ECG was read, whether the finding was recorded on the chart and whether the diagnosis reflected this finding—this is the type of audit that is usually done. In general it is much more difficult—even if standards were agreed upon —to determine, for example, whether and how the health worker explored the patient's anxiety with respect to his or her pain, and whether and how the health worker helped the patient with his or her anxiety.

Measures of so-called patient "compliance" with the health worker's instructions and measures of the patient's satisfaction with care can get at some of these issues, but these are usually much more difficult to implement than the other forms of audit or quality control and therefore relatively little used. It is of interest that when these evaluations are done there is often little correlation between the quality of care as perceived by the patient and the quality determined by professionals based upon review of the medical record.

Dissatisfaction with various measures of the process of care has led to attention to various measures of clinical outcome. But the outcome of care is also difficult to determine, even if one limits the measurement to short-term outcome in specific conditions. Factors such as the extent of disability and the patient's quality of life are difficult to quantify. Further, it is frequently impossible to relate the outcome to any specific element of the process of medical care, and often the outcome may not be related to medical care at all.

Most difficult of all to measure and to relate to a specific form of care is the impact of medical care on the community. Specific effects on specific problems have been determined for certain types of public health measures—such as the effect of fluoridation on tooth decay in children or the effect of immunization on the incidence of specific diseases—and for certain forms of health-care organization—such as the effect of comprehensive care programs on the prevention of rheumatic fever. But these studies can rarely if ever determine the total positive or negative effect of a given procedure or program on the community. Some thought has been given to the development of a broader approach to the evaluation of impact, including in some cases attempts to measure the effects of medical care on the overall quality of life, but most of these ideas are, of course, extremely difficult to implement.

In short, because measuring anything other than the most concretely technical elements of the process and outcome of care remains so difficult, technically related measures are the ones used. The rationale is analogous to that of the inebriated gentleman looking for his money under a street lamp. When asked what he has lost there his response is, "I lost my wallet down the street, but the light is better over here."

In a situation of limited resources, emphasis on one aspect of quality, even if well intentioned, must detract from or drive out other criteria. The result of relying on the definitions and methods used by professional people is an emphasis on the use of technology and a reduction in equity. This shift takes place in such areas as the content, availability and accessibility of care. Examples of the effect on ambulatory care will serve to illustrate the point.

With regard to content, emphasis in the audit on technical performance (as by a checklist of procedures that should be done for a patient with a given diagnosis or presenting problem) may reduce the time and motivation that a health worker has for full exploration of the emotional or social background of the patient's illness and for preventive medicine. It is easy to say piously that the health worker should do both, but if one activity is being audited effectively and the other is being audited ineffectively or not at all, it is clear which activity most health workers will concentrate on; this is another form of what is called "defensive medicine." It is not coincidental that the concentration of attention will be on technical, dependency-producing medicine of exactly the kind that Ivan Illich and other critics find so dysfunctional with respect to health.

Certain kinds of emphasis in audits may affect the availability of ambulatory care when resources are limited. If the audit is concerned only with the quality of the services given to patients who actually see the health worker, or, even worse, with the quality of the services given to patients with specific and easy-to-audit problems, the health worker may use up all of his time in providing such patients with so-called high-quality services, thus decreasing his availability to other people in the community.

Finally and most subtly, an audit emphasis on technical quality may reduce the accessibility of care. Even if cost factors were removed by health insurance with comprehensive coverage and universal entitlement, there are other barriers to care, particularly for the poor and the poorly educated. Problems related to transportation, the impersonality of complex institutions in distant places and the time spent away from children at home or from earning at work—all can be barriers to care. If mechanisms of audit, by their emphasis on high technical quality, cause an increasing number of aspects of care to be shifted out of the neighborhood into large, forbidding, impersonal and distant institutions, it is likely that any improvement in technical quality will be more than overshadowed by the decrease in perceived accessibility for an already disadvantaged group of people.

If professional people continue to carry the major responsibility for assessing the quality of health care, and if they use the methods now being touted for determining that quality, the existing overall maldistribution of power and resources in our society is likely to be exacerbated. This, in all probability, will increase the powerlessness and alienation felt by many people in our communities.

These criticisms of conventional concepts of quality assessment in health care are similar to the criticisms increasingly being leveled at currently fashionable methods of cost-benefit analysis and similar techniques of management. These techniques stress the evaluation of process and of limited measurable types of short-term outcome, often ignoring outcomes that are more difficult to measure in quantitative terms as well as the long-term effects of a given policy. Alfred North Whitehead long ago labeled this type of thinking the "fallacy of misplaced concreteness." The U.S. Department of Defense introduced techniques of this sort under Robert McNamara; the techniques developed a life of their own and were in part responsible for the tragedy of our policy in Vietnam.

The lesson is that if one considers only certain parts of the cost and only certain parts of the results, one may indeed end up with what is seen as efficient short-term management. However, one also may end up with unforeseen costs and long-term results which neither those whom the system is supposed to serve nor those who manage it had intended. It is more important to decide where one is going and whether one needs a train at all than to make the trains run on time.

Those who use these techniques are not unaware of this problem. For example, Charles J. Hitch wrote in 1960 in *The Economics of Defense in the Nuclear Age:*

> Whatever the particular problem, military or civilian, it is fairly obvious that in choosing among alternative means to our ends, we need to scan the ends themselves with a critical eye. New techniques and types of equipment may be extremely efficient in achieving certain aims, but these aims may be the wrong ones —aims that are selected almost unconsciously or at least without sufficient critical thought.

Far too often, those who determine the means thereby continue to determine the ends, while insufficient control of either determination is exercised by those who should be the beneficiaries but are often the victims of the decisions.

The solution, clearly, is to shift the control of assessment of "quality" into the hands of communities, and particularly into the hands of those in communities who are least well served. But several difficulties stand in the way of doing this.

First, communities, and particularly urban communities in the United States, are usually heterogeneous, and it will be difficult to find a commonality of social purose and, therefore, of criteria by which the quality of care is to be measured. Even if that commonality of social purpose is reached, given the power structure of most communities in the United States, the criteria developed by those likely to be chosen to monitor quality may be based on narrow self-interest and thus less likely to stress equity than are professionally determined criteria.

Second, most people in the United States are abysmally ignorant of even the function of their own bodies, not to speak of the intricacies of modern health care in their country. Criteria based in part on ignorance may be self-defeating.

Third, community members may be unwilling to take the time to become knowledgeable or to make considered decisions on community health-care issues unless there is a secondary gain, such as the power to grant jobs. Perhaps they have been conditioned by the long period during which they had no effective method for influencing their health care. Perhaps they are influenced by the need to do more remunerative or pleasurable things with their time. Even affluent people, for example those who have served on the boards of voluntary hospitals, have been taught that health-care institutions are run by professional corporate managers or doctors and that laymen have little to contribute other than philanthropy or lending their prestige to the institution. Such uninterested or cynical nonprofessionals may develop criteria which are less in the community interest than those developed by involved and dedicated professionals.

Fourth, community members often feel intimidated by professional people, either directly or by the threat that the professionals may leave the community rather than work under the control of laymen. Intimidated and anxious nonprofessionals may not be able to set appropriate criteria.

(Incidentally, these and similar difficulties are analogous to those that have made decentralized community control of schools so difficult to implement.)

The response to these difficulties must be neither to give up on the principles nor to deny the problems. A beginning must be made, and with the assignment of responsibility and authority, we believe, will come rapid changes in the ability of community members to deal with these issues. The principle was well stated by Dr. Frantz Fanon with reference to Algeria in his essay "Medicine and Colonialism": "The people who take their destiny into their own hands assimilate the most modern forms of technology at an extraordinary rate." Of course, it was also said earlier and more metaphorically by Mao Tsetung in his essay "On Practice": "If you want to know the taste of a pear, you must change the pear by eating it yourself."

In the American experience, one of the foremost proponents of the principle was Thomas Jefferson: "I know no safe depository of the ultimate powers of the society but the people themselves; and if we think them not enlightened enough to exercise their control with a wholesome discretion, the remedy is not to take it from them but to inform them in their discretion."

The way to begin is by bringing community members into the process of evaluation of quality of care and into decision-making roles whenever there is leverage in the system. As noted earlier, some consumer groups are already engaged in compiling directories of physicians which describe their training and qualifications; others are making similar studies of hospitals from outside them. Community members are already serving on the boards of local Health Systems Agencies, even though their power is still limited and they are still largely controlled directly or indirectly by professionals.

Community members can increasingly be brought into audit committees and onto the boards of trustees of hospitals and other institutions. At first they will have a difficult time standing up to the professionals who dominate these committees and boards, but knowledge and experience can be gained which will bring us closer to true community evaluation and control of the system.

5. *Self-help and Mutual Aid*

According to some observers, there are over one-half million different self-help groups in the United States today. They are by and large consumer-initiated, peer-oriented, problem-centered groups in which the participant is both the helper and the one to be helped. Self-help or mutual-aid groups provide a mechanism whereby individuals in a collective setting with others who face similar life situations can assume responsibility for their own bodies, psyches and behavior and can help others do the same. They are the grass-roots answer to our hierarchical, professionalized society, a society that attempts in so many ways to render impotent the individual, the family, the neighbor. Not only are self-help groups providing desperately needed services, they are returning to the individual a feeling of competence and self-respect and they are forging new links, new connections among people.

Many health-related self-help groups deal with chronic illness and disability. There are, for example, groups for people suffering from obesity, or emphysema, or epilepsy. Groups such as Mended Hearts, Mastectomy, Inc., and Laryngectomy, Inc., help patients adjust to a new physical reality after an operation or other specific treatment for the acute phase of their illness; the laryngectomy group helps its members to improve their speech techniques, and the mastectomy group helps women to face the physical and psychic problems associated with breast loss.

Other self-help groups deal with the many forms of addiction —alcohol, drug and gambling. Groups for families have also recently formed—Al-Anon for spouses of AA members and Alateen for their children, and groups for parents of handicapped children. A recent directory of mutual-help groups in Massachusetts included groups for "parents of twins and multiple births, retarded children, emotionally disturbed children, physically handicapped children, those who face hospitalization, those with leukemia, cystic fibrosis, congenital heart disorders, Down's Syndrome, rubella, spina bifida, Tay-Sachs Disease, cleft palate and/or lip, cerebral palsy, hemophilia, brain injury, and those who are blind or deaf, as well as a group of parents whose child has died."

Self-help groups range from those that provide primary care to those that work in the area of prevention and case finding, from those that do rehabilitative work to those that are concerned with behavior modification. While they provide an opportunity for nonprofessionals to play a helping role and enable individuals to understand and take responsibility for their own bodies and physical states, perhaps their most important contribution is to help to deprofessionalize and demystify medicine in an age of increasing professionalization and technological mystification.

While we see the self-help movement overall as an important and encouraging development, it is often, in our view, a response to the symptoms rather than to the underlying social problems and may in some instances lead to an exacerbation of the deeper problems. Medical self-help groups may, for example, help to perpetuate the basic inequities that characterize our health-care and medical-care system. By relieving some of the pressure on the society to provide preventive services, self-help groups help to perpetuate the disparity between the resources our society devotes to medical care and those it devotes to prevention. Since these groups cannot serve entire segments of the population and frequently serve those who are most actively interested rather than those who are hardest to reach, the self-help movement may be helping to perpetuate the inequality of care in our society by providing care to and thereby neutralizing those who might, out of their dissatisfaction with the system, vocally protest medical inequities. Thus, self-help in the absence of equity may serve to perpetuate inequity.

Furthermore, self-help groups are in many instances permitting professionals to avoid the difficult caring aspects of their professional role and to focus increasingly on its technological aspects. Since self-help groups are not available to everyone in the society and many must still use the professional system to meet their needs, the self-help movement must see as part of its mission the teaching of professionals to work more humanely with their patients. It is also true, however, that while professionals need input from self-help groups, self-help groups need help in technical areas from professionals. Pathways for egalitarian communication must be developed if the system as a whole is to be modified.

Moreover, self-help groups that emphasize individual symptoms and individual problems, such as widowhood, mental retardation or specific medical problems, further fragment individuals, families and communities and further encourage the medicalization of human life. The widow will seek help not from others in her own community but from a group of widows who may have little or nothing in common with one another other than their widowhood. People are encouraged, at the same time, to relate to themselves and to present themselves as a series of symptoms rather than as whole human beings. Self-help groups by their emphasis on specific symptoms and problems emphasize and reinforce those problems rather than making clear that they are an integral part of total human and community life.

Finally, the focusing by self-help groups on individual deviance from the norm places the burden increasingly on that individual to modify his response rather than on the society to modify the conditions which create the response. By singling out the alcoholic, the drug addict, the former mental patient for special help, by placing him in a "therapeutic" environment, society is implicitly stating that he is the problem rather than the victim of the problem. This can turn into simply another of our society's ways of "blaming the victim" rather than attempting to change the conditions that have victimized him. In short, the self-help movement is part of the entire network of human services which by its very existence assumes that the individual must be modified to function within the existing society rather than that the society must be modified to permit and encourage human development.

Thus while we welcome the antielitist, egalitarian character of self-help groups and applaud their efforts at democratizing and demystifying medical care in the United States, we must nevertheless recognize that unless they press for greater equity and build their efforts into existing communities, they, too, are contributing to the fundamental problems of the system.

Nonetheless, the self-help movement, we feel, is a response that stems from an American tradition of mutual aid and antiauthoritarianism and can be built upon in the present and near-future to pave the way for wider popular participation in the field of health in the long run.

6. *Medical Education*

Since physicians to a large extent determine the character of a health-care and medical-care system, a new breed of physician will be required for the successful establishment of a national health service. Since over half the cost of medical education is already borne by the federal government in one way or another, medical schools are vulnerable to pressure for change, and there are a number of areas in which change can be brought about.

Recruitment and selection of students. There are already 45,000 applicants for the 15,000 first-year-class positions in U.S. medical schools. It is estimated that some 40,000 of these applicants are fully qualified to enter medical school—that is, they have the intellectual and emotional capacity to complete the course of study, to pass the licensure examinations and to practice medicine. Medical-school admission committees will therefore be required to make arbitrary choices among the two or more qualified applicants each school has for each of its positions.

In recent years these committees have paid lip service to seeking candidates with personal qualities that might predict their entering primary care in areas now underserved, but the criteria used to pinpoint those qualities are poorly developed. Indeed, one of the few well-accepted correlations of applicant characteristics with post-medical-school performance is that students with the highest undergraduate grade averages are less likely to practice primary care. Yet each year students with the highest academic averages are selected over students with other qualifications for admission to medical schools. Furthermore, over the past decade, although there have been steady increases in the percentage of women in medical schools and (until 1976–77) in the percentage of minority students, the social-class distribution of medical students has changed very little.

Where there have been special efforts to selectively admit students from minority or disadvantaged backgrounds into medical education, these efforts have been frustrated in many different ways. Judicial barriers have been raised against what have been viewed as quota systems favoring minorities, on the grounds of discrimination against the majority students. Even when special efforts continue to be made to seek such students, the fundamental criteria of academic excellence are usually used in choosing among them. This combined with the reluctance of the faculty to change any of its "standards," particularly in the preclinical sciences, leads even after admission to selective weeding out of students who may have qualities that might make them excellent physicians but are not the elite of the elite in terms of academic achievement.

There is no suggestion here that students unqualified to be doctors by any reasonable criteria be admitted to medical school or retained after admission. The argument is that among the 40,000 applicants who are qualified—and the tens of thousands more who are qualified but who do not even bother to apply if their undergraduate grades are not among the very highest—choices should begin to be made on other grounds: grounds of demonstrated interest in serving other people; grounds of special sensitivity to the needs of cultural and ethnic groups who have few physicians who are particularly sensitive to their needs; and on the grounds of conscious increase in equity.

A reconstructed health-care and medical-care system would have many more places for doctors with caring qualities, who can deal with the technological problems raised in primary care but not make technology, rather than care, the focus of their professional lives. And an educational system which produces graduates who reach the peak of their professional lives some 30 years after their selection must begin to plan for the needs of the health- and medical-care system which will be in place in the twenty-first century.

Educational goals and methods. Not only must the mix of medical students be changed but the nature of their education must also be markedly altered. Much of the first two years of medical education is devoted to theoretical training in basic science which is of little direct relevance to the practice of medicine. Much of the last two years of medical education is devoted to education around desperately ill hospitalized patients with problems requiring tertiary care, rather than work with ambulatory patients requiring primary care. Furthermore, much of the socialization in medical school leads students to look upon human beings as objects for study rather than as persons with whom they must work collaboratively to solve problems. Students come to reject as "imaginary" or unworthy of their highly skilled attention those problems for which they can offer no technological fix. They think of themselves as a specially privileged class.

Changing these patterns will be extremely difficult, but there are ways to begin. Students can be brought together with patients, families and communities in a caring, nontechnological role from the beginning of their medical education. The technical elements of medical education can be taught as adjuncts to the basic training in ambulatory patient care. Small parts of the training may have to take place around inpatients in order that the full range of reversible illness which the doctor may see in ambulatory care is presented to the student, but it should be made clear that this is a minor but unavoidable part of their training. Above all, role models of humane, caring doctors must be found with whom the students can identify.

Furthermore, so long as many students are required to pay large amounts for their education (even though those payments are a fraction of the total cost) and for their living expenses during it, there will be an incentive to later "make up for it" by practicing medicine in ways that will maximize income. If, on the other hand, education required no out-of-pocket expenses for tuition and, in addition, a stipend were given for living expenses, the student would graduate feeling himself to be in society's debt rather than society's creditor.

Beyond medical school, all the other societies we have studied limit severely the number of specialist training positions. In the United States the number of positions is largely dependent on the desires of the staff of the particular hospital for the prestige—and the services—provided by house staff training. The number of specialty training programs in the United States, particularly in the surgical specialties, will have to be markedly reduced and postgraduate training in primary care markedly expanded. The services previously provided by house officers in hospitals can be turned over to nurses or to physicians' assistants, almost certainly with net benefit to the patient.

Little of this can be accomplished, however, without removing medical education and postgraduate training from their current control respectively by the Association of American Medical Colleges and by the American Medical Association and the specialty boards. The fact that so much of this training is financed by public funds provides a powerful lever for taking the decision-making out of the hands of these special-interest groups and putting it under public control. While real change in education will require real changes in the models from which students learn, in the short run progress can be made toward equity, provision of physicians in a community context and emphasis on health and on humane care.

In sum, the questions we must ask ourselves about the graduates of our medical schools are the same questions recently posed by the director-general of the World Health Organization at the centenary celebration of the faculty of medicine of the University of Geneva:

> Society, which, after all, foots the bill for all that happens in health, expects us to prepare doctors to fulfil a social purpose in response to the health needs and demands of the community which they are going to serve. The medical school is an integral

part of society, an instrument which should prepare for work *in* and *for* society. . . .

To this end we must arrange an educational program which prepares [graduates] for that role. To do this we have to ask a few searching questions:

Do the graduates think and behave in terms of "health" rather than of "disease"? That is to say, do they apply techniques of prevention and health promotion and not only those of cure and rehabilitation?

Do the graduates think and behave in terms of family and community, rather than in terms of the individual sick patient?

Do the graduates think and behave in terms of membership of a health team consisting of doctors, nurses, and other health workers as well as social scientists and others?

Do the graduates think and behave in terms of making the best and most effective use of the financial and material resources available?

Do the graduates think and behave in terms of their country's patterns of health and disease, and the relevant priorities?

7. *Responsibility to the People of Other Countries*

In these short-term recommendations we must not neglect broader questions of equity and justice, community, health and care among the peoples of the world. For the people of our country to have relatively abundant medical care (not to speak of an abundance of food, clothing, shelter and other necessities of life), however inequitably distributed, while the people of many other countries have little medical care and indeed little of anything but hunger, illness and despair, cannot in our view lead to the fulfillment of our goals. The injustice, the immorality, the ethical bankruptcy of such a situation—and its self-defeating nature—are to us clear on its face, although Garrett Hardin and others would argue that sharing our substance with others is to destroy ourselves by bringing too many people into the "lifeboat." In our view we destroy ourselves by *not* attempting to help those barely clinging to the gunwales.

That we need to help—or, in the short run, not do further harm—is to us clear, but how to accomplish it is less clear. Certainly we must do the obvious things: stop stealing resources (in the form of personnel and profits) from other societies; stop selling inappropriate practices (such as the profitable sale of infant formula by persuading mothers in poor countries to abandon breast-feeding); and start shifting massive amounts of resources in the opposite direction. The UN has urged that wealthy countries contribute at least 1 percent of their GNP to poorer countries. It is shameful that at present we contribute only one-quarter of 1 percent of our GNP to foreign aid while Sweden, for example, contributes close to 1 percent. But even if we contributed this much or more, direct unilateral transfer of these resources might in the short run increase dependence and in the long run increase human misery.

Again, some lessons from China may be relevant. China has taken the position that it will not attempt to export its own methods, but, if a country requests it, will attempt to help that country do those things it wishes to do, whether that entails training barefoot doctors or building a railroad. Canada, through the International Development Research Center, is attempting in similar ways to be guided by the wishes of the people of the recipient countries.

Even the World Health Organization, after decades of building "centers of excellence" based on methods used by industrialized countries, in developing countries which could spend less than a dollar a person per year on all health services, has begun to recognize that such efforts decrease equity, and probably decrease overall health. WHO, as exemplified by recent decisions including the publication of a book entitled *Health by the People*, is beginning to move in the direction of providing aid that emphasizes self-reliance and mass participation.

The United States, by sharing its abundance through international agencies that accept this principle, could be instrumental in helping to make possible the assertion of a right to health care and medical care in other countries as well as in the United States.

The Opposition to a Right to Health Care

A number of arguments are often made in opposition to the concept of a societally guaranteed right to health care and medical care, or to its expression in a national health service. There is merit in cataloging some of these arguments and indicating the nature of our responses to them.

1. A number of economists and other analysts, Milton Friedman being the prototypical example, suggest exactly the opposite course. Their recommendation is that medicine be put back into the marketplace by removing most if not all requirements for medical education and licensure and allowing anyone who wishes to do so to enter practice or open a health center or hospital. The "law of supply and demand" would produce the kind of medical care people want, force down medical-care prices and redistribute medical-care resources. People, the argument goes, would then have free choice, the "good" and "efficient" doctors and faculties would be encouraged and the "bad" and "inefficient" driven out by lack of customers.

This is the exact antithesis of regionalized planning, the antithesis of community organization of care. If one objects to the further erosion of equity which would be the obvious result of such a proposal, the further suggestion is made that vouchers, or even cash, should be given to the poor so that they too can purchase medical care in the marketplace. We reject this proposal for medical-care organization on the grounds—using the same economists' frame of reference—that medicine is a field characterized by scarce resources, imperfect information on the nature of the product, and monopolistic practice, all of which are classically recognized—even by the defenders of the marketplace—to contravene the effective use of the free market. Chipping away at some of these characteristics—*e.g.,* by providing more information to health-care consumers about the training of their doctors—is certainly valuable, but is unlikely to change the basic conditions.

2. A more socially acceptable form of argument is to accept the premise that there is indeed a basic right to health care, but to allege that, since it is economically impossible to provide the "best available" medical care to everyone in a society, the most the right can imply is guaranteed access to some "decent minimum" of health care. Charles Fried, professor of law at Harvard, for example, reaches the following conclusions in a recent article:

1. To say there is a right to health care does not imply a right to equal access, a right that whatever is available to any shall be available to all.

2. The slogan of equal access to the best health care available is just that, a dangerous slogan which could be translated into reality only if we submitted either to intolerable government controls on medical practice or to a thoroughly unreasonable burden of expense.

3. There is sense to the notion of a right to a decent standard of care for all, dynamically defined, but still not dogmatically equated with the best available.

4. We are far from affording such a standard to many of our citizens and that is profoundly wrong.

5. One of the major sources of the exaggerated demands for equality are the pretensions, inflated claims, inefficiencies, and guild-like, monopolistic practices of the health professions.

These conclusions lead Fried into a number of what he calls "practical proposals." Among them is the assuring of each person of "a certain amount of money to purchase medical services as he chooses." There is no notion in the analysis that the right to health care implies equal access and is a step toward equity—in fact, there is an explicit statement that the right to health care has nothing to do with equal access. And there appears to be no consideration of the idea that the ability of some to purchase more or better medical care in the marketplace may, in the face of limited total resources, lead to a denial of the right to adequate—not to speak of equivalent or optimal

—health care to others. In short the argument that the right to health care implies no more than the right to some minimum standard, while others in the society, whatever their relative need for care, can purchase all they want, appears to us in essence a negation of and an argument against the right.

If one believes, as we do, that equity and justice is the foundation and the goal of a society, the only way of approaching that goal in an inequitable and unjust society is to demand that those who now have least will in the future have most access to the best that the society can offer. It is not simply a matter of "equality" of access to the best: The poorest in the United States are also the sickest, and their needs for medical care are far greater than those of the wealthy; thus even equality of access to the best is inherently discriminatory. What we face is a matter of equity, and equity demands redistributive justice, for health care as well as for the other resources of the society.

3. A third argument denies the existence of a right to health care and is much more directly based on the special interests of those who own, control or otherwise profit from the present system. A right to health care, one form of this argument states, implies onerous duties for doctors or other health workers and it is immoral, illegal or both to infringe on the rights of doctors and other health-care workers by dictating where they shall practice and what methods they shall use. This argument was sharply stated in 1971 in an article in the *New England Journal of Medicine* by Dr. Robert Sade:

> The concept of medical care as the patient's right is immoral because it denies the most fundamental of all rights, that of a man to his own life and the freedom of action to support it. Medical care is neither a right nor a privilege: it is a service that is provided by doctors and others to people who wish to purchase it. It is the provision of this service that a doctor depends upon for his livelihood, and is his means of supporting his own life. If the right to health care belongs to the patient, he starts out owning the services of a doctor without the necessity of either earning them or receiving

them as a gift from the only man who has the right to give
them: the doctor himself.

This argument by Dr. Sade against a right to health care has
been reprinted and distributed to doctors and others by medical
societies in the United States.

The argument neglects the fact that over half of the costs of
medical education and some 40 percent of the costs of health
services in the United States are publicly financed. It also neglects the fact that restrictions on the number of medical students and on licensing create a near monopoly. The principle
should be made clear in the United States, as it has been made
clear in other countries, that accepting large quantities of public
funds implies a significant obligation to the society. Perhaps
morality or legality requires that some of these demands be
made of those who enter medical school from now on rather
than imposed *ex post facto,* but from a societal viewpoint the
demands surely must be made.

A more socially acceptable form of the same self-serving
argument states that any significant restriction on profit-making, on earnings or on "clinical judgment" will interfere with
the effectiveness or the efficiency of the system. There is no
evidence, to our knowledge, which supports this contention.
The experience of other countries and our own experience with
well-run public institutions like the Tennessee Valley Authority
indicate that public institutions can be run as or more effectively and efficiently as private ones, and of course serve other
social goals as well.

4. A fourth form of the argument against a right to medical care, and therefore against a national health service, is that
the vast majority of professional medical care is useless or
dangerous, and since one should not have it, there is no inherent
right to it. The viewpoint is stated most explicitly by Ivan Illich,
but many other recent analysts state arguments about the "limits of medicine" which can be used to support the same view.

In our view, the argument that medical care is useless is
vastly overstated. There is evidence, for example, from studies

on the impact of prenatal care on infant mortality in New York City and Denver and on the impact of comprehensive health-care centers on the incidence of rheumatic fever in Baltimore, that medical care can make a substantial difference in outcome. Moreover, medical-care services for the "worried well" and the sick are also important to their comfort and quality of life. Illich is of course correct that there is much that is useless and dangerous in medicine and these elements should be actively constrained and eliminated; but to argue against equitable access to the useful aspects on the grounds that some of the elements are useless is to us a socially irresponsible argument.

An even more pernicious form of this argument is based on the indisputable fact that the health of an individual may depend more on life-style than on medical care. But it does not follow, as many of those who seek to cut tax-supported services argue, that we should therefore devote fewer resources to medical care. What is needed is more effective use of our resources both to make the appropriate societal changes so that individual life-styles can change and to provide appropriate medical care for those who are sick.

5. Finally, there are those who agree that equitable access to health care and medical care is a right, but argue that a national health service would be too complex and too bureaucratic a mechanism through which to achieve it. Our response is that an attempt to provide this access through an insurance reimbursement mechanism has led—and a national health insurance mechanism would further lead—to complexities and bureaucratic superstructures that could be avoided by direct service provision. While a national health service would certainly pose new problems, it would at least bypass the enormous costs of billing, payment, and audit necessary for an insurance program and eliminate some of the temptations for overutilization, overbilling, and gross fraud inherent in reimbursement, whether to the patient or to the provider. In many ways, a national health service will be simpler to decentralize, administer, and control than will national health insurance.

Conclusions

While the experience of our own and other societies demonstrates that the nature of a society's health-care and medical-care system is in large measure determined by its political, economic, social and cultural history, the system can also be a force for change. Because health care and medical care are often seen as making the difference between life and death, they are regarded in many societies as necessities and therefore as basic human rights. The U.S. health-care and medical-care system, from almost every point of view, is failing to meet its responsibilities in the protection and promotion of health and in the provision of humane, competent and efficient care. It is therefore an opportune moment to raise questions about the fundamental purposes of medicine—as one of the service systems of a society—and to attempt to restructure medical care both to better meet both its traditional goals and to serve as a leading edge in moving toward broader social goals.

The task will not be easy. Forces that stand to lose much in power, prestige and profit by any significant changes in the organization of care will condemn and will resist with grim determination any attempt at structural change. Furthermore, since patients are often deeply dependent on physicians and on medical-care institutions, patients will be enlisted as allies in resisting change. Medicine is in some ways a microcosm, a model for the barriers to change in the entire society. But the severe crisis in which medicine finds itself, the fact that it is widely regarded as a necessity rather than a luxury, and some of its traditions of humane and dedicated service make it an arena in which change can begin.

The long-term end—and, more important, means to other ends—of a national health service will not be achieved quickly or easily, and perhaps can never be fully realized without fundamental changes in the society of which it is a part. But by learning from the experiences of other countries and by keeping our goals clearly in mind, we can begin to take steps now that will lead us closer both to changes in the health-care and medical-care system and in the society it serves.

A century ago the distinguished pathologist Rudolf Virchow argued that physicians should be the "natural advocates for the poor." The time has come in the United States to organize a system of care—and to help change the society that surrounds it—so that Virchow's vision of medicine and of the role of those who work within it can become a reality, so that health workers can join those they serve in fostering a healthy state, one with greater equity, community, health and care for all.

BIBLIOGRAPHIC NOTES

Since this book has been written primarily for the general reader, these notes have been prepared in an effort to make them useful to the generalist—as contrasted with the specialist—in seeking further material on the various topics covered. We have therefore concentrated on citing books and articles, particularly recent ones, which may provide the reader with a broader view of health care and medical care in the United States and in other countries and which themselves include primary references if the reader wishes to pursue the topic in greater depth. Primary references have been cited where they have been quoted extensively or where we feel the primary material to be of particular interest.

Introduction

Alexis de Tocqueville's analysis, *Democracy in America,* was originally written in 1834; a recent English translation was published in 1969 by Doubleday Anchor Books (Garden City, N.Y.). Gunnar Myrdal analyzed race relations in the United States in *An American Dilemma* (1944; paperback ed., New York: Pantheon Books, 1944); his description of the contemporary United States may be found in *Against the Stream: Critical Essays on Economics* (New York: Vintage Books, 1975), pp. 266–92.

The concept "blaming the victim" has been forcefully analyzed by William Ryan in *Blaming the Victim* (New York: Vintage Books, 1971). Norman Bethune's "Wounds" is reprinted in Joshua S. Horn, *Away with All Pests* (New York: Monthly Review Press, 1969), pp. 184–86.

Thomas McKeown's analysis of the factors involved in the fall in death rates in England and Wales is presented in *The Role of Medicine: Dream, Mirage, or Nemesis?* (London: Nuffield Provincial Hospitals Trust, 1976). The phenomenon is also discussed by Ivan Illich in *Medical Nemesis: The Expropriation of Health* (New York: Pantheon Books, 1976).

Medical-care services, including those for the "worried well," are discussed by Sidney Garfield in "The Delivery of Medical Care," *Scientific American* 222 (April 1970): 15–23.

A more detailed discussion of the ways in which the individual's social role and perceptions determine choice of goals may be found in Victor W. Sidel, "Quality for Whom? Effects of Professional Responsibility for Quality of Health Care on Equity," *Bulletin of the New York Academy of Medicine* 52 (January 1976): 164–76.

The ethical basis for equity in medical care has been discussed in a large number of recent publications. An example is *Ethics and Health Policy,* edited by Robert Veatch and Roy Branson (Cambridge, Mass.: Ballinger Publishing Co., 1976), particularly the chapters by Outka, Fletcher, Green and Veatch. A more general analysis of equity as a societal goal is presented by John Rawls in *A Theory of Justice* (Cambridge, Mass.: Harvard University Press, 1971). Some of the barriers to achievement of equity in medical care are discussed by Charles E. Lewis, Rashi Fein, and David Mechanic, *A Right to Health: The Problem of Access to Primary Medical Care* (New York: John Wiley & Sons, 1976); Ronald Andersen, Joanna Lion, and Odin W. Anderson, *Equity in Health Services: Empirical Analyses in Social Policy* (Cambridge, Mass.: Ballinger Publishing Co., 1975); Rashi Fein, "On Achieving Access and Equity in Health Care," *Milbank Memorial Fund Quarterly* 50 (October 1972): Part 2: 157–90; and Odin W. Anderson, *Health Care: Can There Be Equity? The United States, Sweden, and England* (New York: John Wiley & Sons, 1972).

The problems of strengthening community life within a highly urbanized society have also been widely discussed. Among the many excellent analyses are Lewis Mumford, *The City in History* (New York: Harcourt Brace Jovanovich, 1961); Jane Jacobs, *The Death and Life of Great American Cities* (New York: Vintage Books, 1961); *Cities: A Scientific American Book* (New York: Alfred A. Knopf, 1967); Herbert J. Gans, *People and Plans: Essays on Urban Problems and Solutions* (New York: Basic Books, 1968); and E. F. Schumacher, *Small Is Beautiful: A Study of Economics As If People Mattered* (New York: Harper & Row, 1974). Aspects of the relationship of health care to community life have been explored in C. A. Doxiadis, "The Inhuman City," in Gordon Wolstenholme and Maeve O'Connor, eds., *Health of Mankind* (London: J. & A. Churchill, 1967); John C. Norman, ed., *Medicine in the Ghetto* (New York: Appleton-Century-Crofts, 1969); and Amasa B. Ford, *Urban Health in America* (New York: Oxford University Press, 1976).

The definition of health and its relationship to health care are analyzed in René Dubos, *Mirage of Health: Utopias, Progress and Biological Change* (Garden City, N.Y.: Doubleday Anchor Books, 1961); Lester Breslow, "A Quantitative Approach to the World Health Organization Definition of Health: Physical, Mental and Social Well-Being," *International Journal of Epidemiology* 1 (Winter 1972): 347–55; Mervyn Susser, "Ethical Components in the Definition of Health," *International Journal of Health Services* 4 (Summer 1974): 539–48; Marc Lalonde, *A New Perspective on the Health of Canadians* (Ottawa: Government of Canada, April 1974); and in McKeown, *Role of Medicine,* and Illich, *Medical Nemesis.*

The caring component of medicine is discussed in Jan Howard and

Anselm L. Strauss, eds., *Humanizing Health Care* (New York: John Wiley & Sons, 1975); in Garfield, "Delivery of Medical Care"; and in the many books and articles cited in the notes for Chapter 1, section 1, below.

Chapter 1. Progress and Problems

Section 1

The number of recent books and articles criticizing aspects of U.S. health care and medical care defies enumeration, not to speak of citation. Those we have listed cover a wide range of critical points of view. Recent general descriptions and analyses of the problems may be found in Rosemary Stevens, *American Medicine and the Public Interest* (New Haven, Conn.: Yale University Press, 1971); *Life and Death and Medicine: A Scientific American Book* (San Francisco: W. H. Freeman & Co., 1973); John G. Freymann, *The American Health Care System: Its Genesis and Trajectory* (New York: Medcom Press, 1974); Spencer Klaw, *The Great American Medicine Show: The Unhealthy State of U.S. Medical Care* (New York: Viking Press, 1975); and John H. Knowles, ed., *Doing Better and Feeling Worse: Health in the United States* (New York: W. W. Norton & Co., 1977). Analyses from economic points of view may be found in Victor R. Fuchs, *Who Shall Live? Health, Economics, and Social Choice* (New York: Basic Books, 1974), and Rashi Fein, "Some Health Policy Issues: One Economist's View," *Public Health Reports* 90 (September–October 1975): 387–92. Recent sociological analyses, again from differing points of view, have been made by Eliot Freidson, *Profession of Medicine: A Study of the Sociology of Applied Knowledge* (New York: Dodd, Mead & Co., 1970); David Mechanic, *The Growth of Bureaucratic Medicine: An Inquiry into the Dynamics of Patient Behavior and the Organization of Medical Care* (New York: John Wiley & Sons, 1976); and Howard B. Waitzkin and Barbara Waterman, *The Exploitation of Illness in Capitalist Society* (Indianapolis: Bobbs-Merrill Co., 1974). Closely related are political analyses such as those by Robert R. Alford, *Health Care Politics: Ideological and Interest Group Barriers to Reform* (Chicago: University of Chicago Press, 1975), and Theodore Marmor, *The Politics of Medicare* (Chicago: Aldine Pub-

lishing Co., 1973). The institutions of U.S. medicine have been critically analyzed by the Health Policy Advisory Committee (Health-
PAC) in Barbara and John H. Ehrenreich, eds., *The American Health
Empire: Power, Profits, and Politics* (New York: Vintage Books,
1971), and in David Kotelchuck, ed., *Prognosis Negative: Crisis in the
Health Care System* (New York: Vintage Books, 1970). Critics who
raise basic questions about the efficacy of medical care include Ivan
Illich, *Medical Nemesis*, cited above, and Rick J. Carlson, *The End
of Medicine* (New York: John Wiley & Sons, 1975). A Marxist analysis has been provided by Vicente Navarro in *Medicine Under Capitalism* (New York: Prodist, 1976). And the personal points of view of
two participant-observers attempting to change different aspects of
the system are presented by Fitzhugh Mullan, *White Coat, Clenched
Fist: The Political Education of an American Physician* (New York:
Macmillan Co., 1976), and George Silver, *A Spy in the House of
Medicine* (Germantown, Md.: Aspen Systems Corp., 1976). One of
the few books defending the existing structure of the U.S. health-care
system is Harry Schwartz, *The Case for American Medicine* (New
York: David McKay Co., 1972).

The articles on medicine in the January 1970 issue of *Fortune* were
reprinted in *Our Ailing Medical System* (New York: Harper & Row,
1970), and the statement by Department of Health, Education and
Welfare Secretary Elliot Richardson was made in testimony before
the Subcommittee on Health of the Committee on Labor and Public
Welfare, U.S. Senate, February 22–23, 1971, part I, pp. 72–5. *The
New York Times* articles on incompetence among physicians and
other dangers of medical care, written by Boyce Rensberger and Jane
E. Brody, ran from January 26 through January 30, 1976.

Data on death rates and life expectancy in the United States are
collected by the National Center for Health Statistics of the Department of Health, Education and Welfare and published annually in
Vital Statistics of the United States. Summaries and analyses of these
and other statistical data used in this chapter may be found in *Health
United States 1975,* published in 1976 by the National Center as
DHEW Publication no. (HRA) 76–1232. Data for 1975 may be found
in the statement by the director of the National Center for Health
Statistics before the Senate Health Subcommittee on March 31, 1977.

The data suggesting the recent fall in the death rate from coronary
heart disease are analyzed by Gina Bari Kolata and Jean L. Marx in
"Epidemiology of Heart Disease: Searches for Causes," *Science* 194

(October 29, 1976): 509–12. They state that "some epidemiologists would like to see the trend continue for a few more years in order to be sure it is not a statistical quirk," but that "most believe the trend is real." More recent data were reported by the National Center for Health Statistics in the testimony cited above, and suggest that the trend is continuing.

Section 2

A more detailed comparison, "The Mortality of Swedish and U.S. White Males, 1969–1971," is presented by R. F. Tomasson in the *American Journal of Public Health* 66 (October 1976): 968–74. Victor Fuchs's analysis of the interstate differences in death rates can be found on pp. 52–4 of *Who Shall Live?* also cited above, and the variations in infant and postneonatal mortality rates of deaths from accidents, suicide and homicide in the United Kingdom with those in the United States were reported in a July 1976 mimeographed draft report, "National Health Planning Guidelines," prepared by the Department of Health, Education and Welfare for use by the staffs of local health systems agencies. The comparison of infant mortality in poverty and nonpoverty areas may be found in "Selected Vital and Health Statistics in Poverty and Nonpoverty Areas of 19 Large Cities, United States, 1969–71," ser. 21, no. 26, of *Vital and Health Statistics,* published by the National Center for Health Statistics as DHEW Publication no. (HRA) 76–1904. The data on maternal mortality and comparative death rates were presented by Robert Maxwell in table 5 of *Health Care: The Growing Dilemma* (New York: McKinsey & Co., 1975); his sources were the *World Health Statistics Reports* published regularly by the World Health Organization.

The article identifying preventable medical conditions is David D. Rutstein and others, "Measuring the Quality of Medical Care: A Clinical Method," *New England Journal of Medicine* 294 (March 11, 1976): 582–8.

The estimate of incidence of hepatitis associated with blood transfusions is given in *Forward Plan for Health, FY 1977–81,* DHEW Publication no. (OS) 76–50024, August 1975. Richard Titmuss's cross-national study of blood donations can be found in *The Gift Relationship* (New York: Pantheon Books, 1971).

The official report of the World Health Organization collaborative study is Robert Kohn and Kerr L. White, eds., *Health Care: An*

International Study (New York: Oxford University Press, 1976). A summary of the report may be found in the August 1975 issue of *Scientific American* (Kerr L. White, "International Comparisons of Medical Care," 233: 17–25).

The data on chronic illness and disability and the height differences in the United States between poor and nonpoor U.S. children were collected by the National Center for Health Statistics, reported in *Vital and Health Statistics,* and summarized in *Health United States 1975,* cited above.

The inadequate diet of millions of Americans was documented by the Citizens Board of Inquiry into Hunger and Malnutrition in the United States and was published in Atlanta in 1973 by the board and by the Southern Regional Council in the report *Hunger U.S.A. Revisited.* The study demonstrating the elimination of growth differences related to social class in Sweden was performed by Gunilla Lindgren, "Height, Weight and Menarche in Swedish Urban School Children in Relation to Socio-economic and Regional Factors," *Annals of Human Biology* 3 (November 1976): 501–28.

The data on the number of young men found unqualified for military service were presented in the report of the President's Task Force on Manpower Conservation, *One-Third of a Nation* (Washington, D.C.: U.S. Government Printing Office, January 1, 1964).

Section 3

Detailed data on the fiscal aspects of health and medical care in the United States may be found in *Medical Care Expenditures, Prices, and Costs: Background Book,* published by the Department of Health, Education and Welfare, Social Security Administration, as DHEW Publication no. (SSA) 75–11909, and in *Health United States 1975,* cited above. Later data were published by Robert M. Gibson and Marjorie Smith Mueller, "National Health Expenditures, Fiscal Year 1976," *Social Security Bulletin,* April 1977, pp. 3–22.

The changes in the number of laboratory tests performed for patients with specific illnesses were determined by Anne A. Scitovsky and Nelda McCall and published in *Changes in the Costs of Treatment of Selected Illnesses, 1951–1964–1971,* published by the Department of Health, Education and Welfare, Public Health Service, as DHEW Publication no. (HRA) 77–3161. The van der Sande experience is in Daniel Schorr, *Don't Get Sick in America* (Nashville, Tenn.: Aurora

Publishers, 1970). Annual data on private health insurance in the United States are published by the Health Insurance Institute, New York, as the *Source Book of Health Insurance Data.* The profits of drug companies, insurance companies and nursing-home owners are discussed in Kotelchuck, ed., *Prognosis Negative,* cited above. A detailed analysis of the drug industry is given in Martin Silverman and Philip R. Lee, *Pills, Profits, and Politics* (Berkeley: University of California Press, 1974), and of the nursing-home industry in Mary Adelaide Mendelson, *Tender Loving Greed* (New York: Vintage Books, 1975).

The data on the incomes for physicians and for male salaried workers and on the amounts spent on alcohol, tobacco, etc., are given in *The Statistical Abstract of the United States 1976,* prepared by the Bureau of the Census of the United States. The comparative incomes of health workers are discussed by Vicente Navarro in *Medicine Under Capitalism,* cited above.

Section 4

Changes in the leading causes of death in the United States and their implications are analyzed by William H. Glazier in the "Task of Medicine," *Scientific American* 228 (April 1973): 13–17. Data on preventable conditions are presented in *Forward Plan For Health FY 1977–81,* cited above, and *Forward Plan For Health FY 1978–82.* Infant mortality in New York City was analysed by David Kessner and others, *Infant Death: An Analysis by Maternal Risk and Health Care* (Washington, D.C.: Institute of Medicine, National Academy of Sciences, 1973), and data on the rate of physical examinations for children under the age of 17 were gathered by the National Health Interview Survey and summarized in *Health United States 1975,* cited above.

Section 5

A recent detailed and comprehensive description of the United States health-care and medical-care system, with an extensive bibliography, may be found in Steven Jonas and others, *Health Care Delivery in the United States* (New York: Springer Publishing Co., 1977). Detailed data on distribution of hospitals and health workers, on physicians' visits and on health problems may be found in *Health*

United States 1975, cited above. Detailed data on the geographic distribution of doctors, nurses and other health workers are presented in *Health Resources Statistics,* issued annually by the National Center for Health Statistics; the most recent volume, for 1975, is DHEW Publication no. (HRA) 76–1509.

An analysis of barriers to health care for the poor was made by L. Bergner and A. S. Yerby, "Low Income and Barriers to Use of Health Services," *New England Journal of Medicine* 278 (March 7, 1968): 541–6. The study of teletherapy units in the city of Chicago and the report of the Inter-Society Commission were discussed by Spencer Klaw in *The Great American Medicine Show,* cited above.

Section 6

The data on X-ray examinations, drug use and reactions, surgery and the competence of physicians in the United States were presented in the series of articles in *The New York Times* written by Boyce Rensberger and Jane E. Brody and published January 26–30, 1976.

The studies on deferrable surgery were reported by Eugene G. McCarthy and Geraldine W. Widmer, "Effects of Screening by Consultants on Recommended Elective Surgical Procedures," *New England Journal of Medicine* 291 (December 19, 1974): 1331–5. The implications of the study have been disputed, for example, by Ralph Emerson, "Unjustified Surgery: Fact or Myth?" *New York State Journal of Medicine* 76 (March 1976): 454–61. The data on the variations in the rate of surgery in Kansas were presented by Charles E. Lewis, "Variations in the Incidence of Surgery," *New England Journal of Medicine* 281 (October 16, 1969): 880–4. Comparisons between numbers of surgeons and rates of surgery in England and the United States were made by John P. Bunker, "Surgical Manpower," *New England Journal of Medicine* 282 (January 15, 1970): 135–44.

Section 7

Data on the current numbers of health workers in the United States may be found in the annual editions of *Health Resources Statistics,* cited above. Distribution of health workers in 1970 and projections to 1990 were presented in *The Supply of Health Manpower,* DHEW Publication no. (HRA) 75–38. An analysis of the authority of the physician has been presented by Eliot Freidson in *Professional Domi-*

nance: The Social Structure of Medical Care (New York: Atherton Press, 1970), pp. 108–9.

The quotation on the withholding of information is from Ronald J. Glasser, *Ward 402* (New York: Pocket Books, 1974), p. 69.

A discussion of characteristics and roles of health workers can be found in Barbara Ehrenreich and John H. Ehrenreich, "Hospital Workers: Class Conflicts in the Making," and in Carol A. Brown, "Women Workers in the Health Service Industry," published, respectively, in the *International Journal of Health Services* 5, no. 1 (1975): 43–51; no. 2 (1975): 173–84; and in Vicente Navarro, "Women in Health Care," *New England Journal of Medicine* 292 (February 20, 1975): 398–402. A series of articles describing nurse-doctor relationships is presented in Bonnie Bullough and Vern Bullough, eds., *New Directions for Nurses* (New York: Springer Publishing Co., 1971), particularly Leonard I. Stein, "The Doctor-Nurse Game," pp. 129–37. Further analysis of these relationships can be found in Shirley A. Smoyak, "Problems in Interprofessional Relations," *Bulletin of the New York Academy of Medicine* 53 (January–February 1977): 51–9. The quotation describing the alienated worker is taken from Freidson's *Professional Dominance,* p. 144.

Data on the characteristics of U.S. medical students are published regularly in the *Journal of Medical Education* and annually in the medical-education issue of the *Journal of the American Medical Association;* the December 27, 1976, issue gives data for the classes entering and graduating in 1975.

Further material on the development of the "intermediate" categories of health personnel and the issues surrounding their training can be found in the following sources: Donald M. Pitcairn and Daniel Flahault, eds., *The Medical Assistant: An Intermediate Level of Health Care Personnel,* Public Health Paper no. 60 (Geneva: World Health Organization, 1974); Alfred M. Sadler, Jr., Blair L. Sadler, and Ann A. Bliss, *The Physician's Assistant: Today and Tomorrow* (Cambridge, Mass.: Ballinger Publishing Co., 1975); Susan Reverby, "The Sorcerer's Apprentice," in Kotelchuck, ed., *Prognosis Negative,* pp. 215–29, previously cited; Margaret E. Mahoney, "The Future Role of Physicians' Assistants and Nurse Practitioners," in John Z. Bowers and Elizabeth Purcell, eds., *National Health Services: Their Impact on Medical Education and Their Role in Prevention* (New York: Josiah Macy, Jr., Foundation, 1973), pp. 124–42; and Anthony Robbins, "Allied Health Manpower—Solution or Problem?" *New England*

Journal of Medicine 286 (April 27, 1972): 918–23. Examples of studies on their effectiveness and acceptance include Charles E. Lewis and others, "Activities, Events and Outcomes in Ambulatory Patient Care," *New England Journal of Medicine* 280 (March 20, 1969): 645–9; Evan Charney and Harriet Kitzman, "The Child-Health Nurse (Pediatric Nurse Practitioner) in Private Practice: A Controlled Trial," *New England Journal of Medicine* 285 (December 9, 1971): 1353–8; Eugene C. Nelson, Arthur R. Jacobs, and Kenneth G. Johnson, "Patients' Acceptance of Physicians' Assistants," *Journal of the American Medical Association* 228 (April 1, 1974): 63–7; and Lawrence S. Linn, "Patient Acceptance of the Family Nurse Practitioner," *Medical Care* 14 (April 1976): 357–64. Marianne G. Dekker documents "First Doctor Opposition to Physician's Assistants" in *Medical Economics,* September 6, 1976. Warnings that the use of nonphysician personnel to provide primary care is likely to further the two-class nature of medical care in the United States, with the poor cared for by those with less training, were sounded by Milton Terris, "False Starts and Lesser Alternatives," *Bulletin of the New York Academy of Medicine* 53 (January–February 1977): 129–40, and Milton I. Roemer, "Primary Care and Physician Extenders in Affluent Countries," *International Journal of Health Services* 7 (Fall 1977): 545–55.

The decrease in home visits, demonstrated by the National Health Interview Survey, was summarized in *Forward Plan for Health FY 1978–82,* cited above, p. 16.

Section 8

The dehumanization of the U.S. medical-care system is discussed in Jan Howard and Anselm L. Strauss, eds., *Humanizing Health Care* (New York: John Wiley & Sons, 1975), particularly the chapter by H. Jack Geiger, "The Causes of Dehumanization in Health Care and the Prospects for Humanization," pp. 11–36. The study of patient care in a teaching hospital is described in Raymond S. Duff and August B. Hollingshead, *Sickness and Society* (New York: Harper & Row, 1968), p. 277. A discussion of some of the problems of providing medical care to patients with different cultural beliefs about health can be found in Alan Haywood, "The Hot-Cold Theory of Disease: Implications for Treatment of Puerto Rican Patients," *Journal of the American Medical Association* 216 (May 17, 1971): 1153–8, and in

Walsh McDermott, Kurt W. Deuschle, and Clifford R. Barnett, "Health Care Experiment at Many Farms," *Science* 175 (January 7, 1972): 23–31.

Michael Crichton's description of the use of television for remote-control medical care can be found in *Five Patients* (New York: Alfred A. Knopf, 1970), pp. 115–54.

Differences in diagnosis and care based on the social class of the patient have been presented in August Hollingshead and Frederick Redlich, *Social Class and Mental Illness* (New York: John Wiley & Sons, 1958); Barney G. Glazer and Anselm L. Strauss, *Awareness of Dying* (Chicago: Aldine Publishing Co., 1967); David Sudnow, "Dead on Arrival," in Anselm L. Strauss, ed., *Where Medicine Fails* (New Brunswick, N.J.: Transaction Books, 1973), pp. 193–211; and Andrew Twaddle, "Life Values, Life Chances and Life Styles," *Journal of Operational Psychiatry* 5 (Fall/Winter 1973): 13–23.

Ivan Illich's definition of "social iatrogenesis" is from his book *Medical Nemesis,* pp. 41 and 127, previously cited. Irving K. Zola discusses "Medicine as an Institution of Social Control" in Caroline Cox and Adrianne Mead, eds., *A Sociology of Medical Practice* (London: Collier-Macmillan, 1975), pp. 170–85.

Section 9

General aspects of foreign-physician migration to the United States are discussed in Stephen S. Mick, "The Foreign Medical Graduate," *Scientific American* 232 February 1975: 14–21, and Rosemary Stevens, Louis Wolf Goodman, Stephen S. Mick, and June G. Darge, "Physician Migration Reexamined," *Science* 190 (October 31, 1975): 439–42. The impact of physician migration on the donor countries is discussed by Oscar Gish, *Doctor Migration and World Health: The Impact of the International Demand for Doctors on Health Services in Developing Countries* (London: G. Bell & Sons, 1971), and by Hossain A. Ranaghy, Elaine Zeighami, and Bahram Zeighami, "Physician Migration to the U.S.—Foreign Aid for U.S. Manpower," *Medical Care* 14 (June 1976): 502–11. The impact in the United States is discussed by T. D. Dublin, "Foreign Physicians: Their Impact on U.S. Health Care," *Science* 185 (August 2, 1974): 407–14; Robert J. Weiss, Joel C. Kleinman, Ursula C. Brandt, and Dan S. Felsenthal, "The Effect of Importing Physicians—Return to Pre-Flexnerian Standards," *New England Journal of Medicine* 290 (June 27, 1974):

1453–8; and Kathleen N. Williams and Robert H. Brook, "Foreign Medical Graduates and Their Impact on the Quality of Medical Care in the United States," *Milbank Memorial Fund Quarterly* 53 (Fall 1975): 549–81.

Information on the drug-marketing practices of multinational corporations can be found in Milton Silverman, *The Drugging of the Americas* (Berkeley: University of California Press, 1976), and Sanjaya Lall, "Medicines and Multinationals," *Monthly Review* 10 (March 1977): 19–30. The attempt to persuade women in poor countries to adopt bottle-feeding rather than breast-feeding is documented in Ted Greiner, *The Promotion of Bottle Feeding by Multinational Corporations: How Advertising and the Health Professions Have Contributed,* Cornell International Nutrition Monograph no. 2 (Ithaca, N.Y.: Cornell University Program on International Nutritional Development Policy, 1975).

An analysis of the relationship between public health and imperialism, with special reference to the Rockefeller Foundation, can be found in E. Richard Brown, "Public Health in Imperialism: Early Rockefeller Programs at Home and Abroad," *American Journal of Public Health* 66 (September 1976): 897–903.

Introduction to Part 2

Sources on international comparisons of health care and medical care take a number of different forms. Comparative material is often available in articles or books written on one country. We have listed such books under the country with which it is predominantly concerned; for example, Gordon Hyde's book, cited in the USSR chapter, includes comparative material on Great Britain. Other materials specifically attempt to compare services in a defined group of countries: E. Richard Weinerman, *Social Medicine in Eastern Europe* (Cambridge, Mass.: Harvard University Press, 1969); John Fry, *Medicine in Three Societies: A Comparison of Medical Care in the USSR, USA and UK* (New York: American Elsevier Publishing Co., 1970); Odin W. Anderson, *Health Care: Can There Be Equity? The United States, Sweden, and England* (New York: John Wiley & Sons, 1972); Hugh Heilo, *Modern Social Politics in Britain and Sweden: From Relief to Income Maintenance* (New Haven, Conn.: Yale University Press,

1974); Michael Kaser, *Health Care in the Soviet Union and Eastern Europe* (London: Croom Helm, 1976); and Milton Roemer, *Health-Care Systems in World Perspective* (Ann Arbor, Mich.: Health Administration Press, 1976). Other references include brief descriptions of medical care in a number of different countries, often contributed by specialists in those countries: John Fry and W. A. J. Farndale, eds., *International Medical Care: A Comparison and Evaluation of Medical Care Services Throughout the World* (Wallingford, Penn.: Washington Square East Publishers, 1972); I. Douglas-Wilson and Gordon McLachlan, eds., *Health Service Prospects: An International Survey* (Boston: Little, Brown & Co., 1973); John Z. Bowers and Elizabeth Purcell, eds., *National Health Services* (New York: Josiah Macy, Jr., Foundation, 1973); O. Fulcher, *Medical Care Systems: Public and Private Health Coverage in Selected Industrialized Countries* (Geneva: International Labor Office, 1974); J. G. Simanis, *National Health Systems in Eight Countries* (Washington, D.C.: Department of Health, Education and Welfare, Social Security Administration, 1975); and Kenneth Newell, ed., *Health by the People* (Geneva: World Health Organization, 1975).

There are a number of reports of detailed comparative international studies of specific aspects of medical care. Two recent examples are *The Report of the WHO International Collaborative Study of Medical Care Utilization*, cited in the notes for Chapter 1, and Brian Abel-Smith, *Value for Money in Health Services: A Comparative Study* (London: William Heinemann, 1976).

Chapter 2. Sweden—Planned Pluralism

Brief descriptions of the Swedish health-care system may be found in the books by Odin W. Anderson, O. Fulcher, and J. G. Simanis and in the chapter by S. Ake Lindgren in Wilson and McLachan, eds., *Health Service Prospects*, all cited in the notes to the Introduction to Part 2. More detailed descriptions of various aspects of health care in Sweden may be found in Vicente Navarro, *National and Regional Health Planning in Sweden*, published in 1974 as DHEW Publication no. (NIH) 72–240; *Health and Medical Care Services: The County Councils in Sweden* (Stockholm: Federation of Swedish County Councils, 1972); Bengt Mollstedt, *Public Health in Sweden: Health Services, Environmental Hygiene and Health Education* (Stockholm: Swedish

Institute, 1972); Budd Shenkin, "Politics and Medical Care in Sweden: The Seven Crowns Reform," *New England Journal of Medicine* 288 (March 15, 1973): 555–9; a series of articles by Lawrence K. Altman which appeared in the *New York Times* from April to July 1973; and the special health-care issue of *Scandinavian Review* 63 (September 1975), particularly the article by Ragnar Berfenstam and Ray H. Elling, "Regional Planning in Sweden: A Social and Medical Problem," pp. 40–52, from which many of the specific current data were taken. There are a number of comparative studies of aspects of care in Sweden and the United States, including Ronald Andersen, Bjorn Smedby, and Odin W. Anderson, *Medical Care Use in Sweden and the United States: A Comparative Analysis of Systems and Behavior* (Chicago: Center for Health Administration Studies, 1970); Ronald Andersen and Bjorn Smedby, "Changes in Response to Symptoms of Illness in the United States and Sweden," *Inquiry,* Supplement to vol. 12 (June 1975); pp. 116–27; and Egon Jonsson and Duncan Neuhauser, "Hospital Staffing Ratios in the United States and Sweden," *Inquiry,* loc. cit., pp. 128–37.

The vast differences between infant mortality in the United States and Sweden have recently been analyzed by M. J. Smith, "Reflections on Infant Mortality and Nation's Health," *Rocky Mountain Medical Journal* 72 (November 1975): 471–4, and H. M. Wallace and H. Goldstein, "Status of Infant Mortality in Sweden and the United States," *Journal of Pediatrics* 87 (December 1975): 995–1000. Occupational health efforts in Sweden are described in Sven Forssman, *The New Work Environment* (Stockholm: Swedish Institute, 1975).

Articles on recent developments in the Swedish health-care system include James K. Cooper, "Sweden's No-Fault Patient-Injury Insurance," *New England Journal of Medicine* 294 (June 3, 1976): 1268–70; Kristina Berg, "General Practice in Sweden," *Journal of the Royal College of General Practitioners* 25 (April 1975): 305–7; and Gunnar Wennstrom, "The Public Health Planning System in Sweden," in N. T. J. Bailey and M. Thompson, eds., *Systems Aspects of Health Planning* (Amsterdam: North-Holland Publishing Co., 1975).

Chapter 3. Great Britain—Equitable Entitlement

Rosemary Stevens' *Medical Practice in Modern England: The Impact of Specialization and State Medicine* (New Haven, Conn.: Yale University Press, 1966) is one of the best single sources on the history and structure of the British National Health Service. Brief descriptions of the NHS may be found in the books by John Fry, Odin W. Anderson and J. G. Simanis and in chapters by Gordon Forsyth in Wilson and McLachlan, eds., *Health Service Prospects*, A. T. Elder in Fry and Farndale, eds., *International Medical Care*, and Lord Rosenheim in Bowers and Purcell, eds., *National Health Services*, all cited in the notes to the Introduction to Part 2. Ann Cartwright's *Patients and Their Doctors: A Study of General Practice* (London: Routledge & Kegan Paul, 1967) describes the results of a nationwide survey into the attitudes and practices of patients and general practitioners.

A recent review of the history and structure of the NHS, *The British Health Care System*, was written in 1976 by Economic Models Limited of London for the American Medical Association. Quite another point of view is offered by Dr. David Stark Murray, president of the Socialist Medical Association from 1951 to 1970, in *Why a National Health Service? The Part Played by the Socialist Medical Association* (London: Pemberton Books, 1971).

A trenchant description of the role of the GP may be found in M. Marinker, *The Doctor and His Patient* (Leicester: Leicester University Press, 1975), which also includes the apothecary's sign quoted on page 135.

Detailed material on the history of health care and medical care in Britain may be found in Stevens, *Medical Problems in Modern England*, including, on p. 33, the quote on the hospital and the patient; George Rosen, *From Medical Police to Social Medicine: Essays on the History of Health Care* (New York: Science History Publications, 1974); Philip Rhodes, *The Value of Medicine* (London: George Allen & Unwin, 1976); and the section on Britain in Anderson, *Health Care: Can There Be Equity?* cited previously. A detailed description of the development of the English poor laws and of public health in Britain can be found in W. M. Frazer, *A History of English Public Health, 1834–1939* (London: Balliere, Tindall & Cox, 1950). Aneurin Bevan's views on the need for a national health service are presented in his book *In Place of Fear* (New York: Simon & Schuster, 1952).

Ruth Levitt, *The Reorganized National Health Service* (London: Croom Helm, 1976), and Steven Jonas and David Banta, "The 1974 Reorganization of the British National Health Service: An Analysis," *Journal of Community Health* 1 (Winter 1975): 91–105, are excellent descriptions of the 1974 reorganization; the quotation on page 144 is from Levitt, p. 17. The new role for the specialty of community medicine under the reorganization is discussed in Alonzo S. Yerby, *Community Medicine in England and Scotland,* published in 1976 as DHEW Publication no. (NIH) 76–1061. A detailed study of community health councils (including, on p. 21, the quotation on their scope) is provided in Rudolf Klein and Janet Lewis, *The Politics of Consumer Representation: A Study of Community Health Councils* (London: Centre for Studies in Social Policy, 1976).

Julian Tudor Hart's analysis of the "inverse care law" can be found in his chapter in Caroline Cox and Adrianne Mead, eds., *A Sociology of Medical Practice* (London: Collier-Macmillan, 1975), pp. 189–206; his description of the inequities remaining in the NHS can be found on p. 205. A series of official publications on the priorities of the National Health Service, published by Her Majesty's Stationery Office in London in 1976, include *Prevention and Health: Everybody's Business,* prepared jointly by the Health Departments of Great Britain and Northern Ireland, and *Priorities for Health and Personal Social Services in England* and *Sharing Resources for Health in England,* prepared by the Department of Health and Social Security in London. These documents, which recommend major shifts in allocations of resources, are being widely debated in Britain, for example, by the Radical Statistics Health Group in their pamphlet *Whose Priorities?* (1976).

Chapter 4. The Soviet Union—Centralized Socialism

Further general reading on the Soviet health-care system can be found in books by Mark G. Field, a U.S. sociologist: *Doctor and Patient in Soviet Russia* (Cambridge, Mass.: Harvard University Press, 1957) and *Soviet Socialized Medicine: An Introduction* (New

York: Free Press, 1967). A more recent analysis of the Soviet system by Field is his chapter "Health As a 'Public Utility' or the 'Maintenance of Capacity' in Soviet Society" in a book also edited by him, *Social Consequences of Modernization in Communist Societies* (Baltimore: Johns Hopkins University Press, 1976). Gordon Hyde, a British physician, has written a history of Soviet health services and a description of the current system, and has included comparative material on the British system in his book *The Soviet Health Service: A Historical and Comparative Study* (New York: Beekman Publishers, 1974). Vicente Navarro has provided a Marxist critique in his recent book, *Social Security and Medicine in the USSR* (Lexington, Mass.: D.C. Heath and Co., 1977). Brief descriptions of the medical-care system in the USSR may be found in John Fry, *Medicine in Three Societies* and in chapters by John Fry and L. Crane in Fry and Farndale, eds., *International Medical Care* and by Dmitri Venediktov in Wilson and McLachlan, eds., *Health Services Prospects.*

Important historical works, written at a different phase of the development of the Soviet health system and of Soviet society, include Sir Arthur Newsholme and John Adams Kingsbury, *Red Medicine: Socialized Health in Soviet Russia* (Garden City, N.Y.: Doubleday, Doran & Co., 1933), and two books by Henry Sigerist, *Socialized Medicine in the Soviet Union* (New York: W. W. Norton & Co., 1937) and *Medicine and Health in the Soviet Union* (New York: Citadel Press, 1947).

Material published by the World Health Organization on health care and medical care in the USSR includes G. A. Popov's *Principles of Health Planning in the USSR,* Public Health Paper no. 43 (Geneva: WHO, 1971) and *The Training and Utilization of Feldshers in the USSR,* Public Health Paper no. 56 (Geneva: WHO, 1974). Recent Soviet health studies from the Fogarty International Center for Advanced Study in the Health Sciences, National Institutes of Health, Bethesda, Maryland, include M. S. Massell, *Soviet Medicine: A Bibliography of Bibliographies; Urban Emergency Medical Services of the City of Leningrad* (translated from the Russian, 1975); and A. P. Zhuk, *Public Health Planning in the USSR* (translated from the Russian, 1976). Materials published in English by official sources in the USSR include Yuri Lisitsin, *Health Protection in the USSR* (Moscow: Progress Publishers, 1972), and Nikolai Shesternya, *USSR: Health Protection* (Moscow: Novosti Press Agency Publishing House, 1976).

The quotations on health and industrialization are from Hyde, *The Soviet Health Service,* p. 98. Further data on occupational medicine can be found in R. Rapord, "Industrial Health Services in the USSR," *World Health,* March 1969, p. 20.

Additional material on the feldsher may be found in Victor W. Sidel, "Feldshers and 'Feldsherism,'" *New England Journal of Medicine* 278 (April 25 and May 2, 1962): 934–39, 987–92; and in a number of recent WHO publications on health personnel.

The evaluation of pre–World War I Russia is from Sigerist, *Medicine and Health in the Soviet Union,* p. 78. The statements by Lenin on typhus and on lice are in vol. 30 of Lenin's *Collected Works* (London: Lawrence & Wishart, 1965).

Details on current Soviet practices are presented in recent articles in the U.S. medical literature, such as Patrick B. Storey and Russel B. Roth, "Emergency Medical Care in the Soviet Union," *Journal of the American Medical Association* 217 (August 2, 1971): 588–92; Patrick B. Storey, "Continuing Medical Education in the Soviet Union," *New England Journal of Medicine* 285 (August 19, 1971): 437–42; and Roger I. Glass, "A Perspective on Environmental Health in the USSR," *Archives of Environmental Health* 30 (August 1975): 391–5.

Materials citing some of the remaining problems include Zhores Medvedev and Roy Medvedev, *A Question of Madness* (New York: Vintage Books, 1972), and Ludmilla Thorne, "Inside Russia's Psychiatric Jails," *The New York Times Magazine* (June 12, 1977): 26–71, vivid descriptions of the political uses of psychiatry in the Soviet Union; two books on the Soviet Union written by American journalists Robert G. Kaiser, *Russia: The People and the Power* (New York: Pocket Books, 1976), and Hedrick Smith, *The Russians* (New York: Ballantine Books, 1976); and the *Current Digest of the Soviet Press,* published weekly by the American Association for the Advancement of Slavic Studies (from which, for example, comes the translation of the article in *Literaturnaya Gazeta,* September 25, 1974, which refers to the shortage of drugs).

Chapter 5. The People's Republic of China—Mass Mobilization

General descriptions of China's health-care and medical-care system are to be found in Joshua Horn, *Away with All Pests... an English Surgeon in People's China, 1954–1969* (New York: Monthly Review Press, 1969); Mark Selden, *China: Revolution and Health,* Health-PAC Bulletin no. 47 (1972); Peter Wilenski, *The Delivery of Health Services in the People's Republic of China* (Ottawa: International Development Research Centre, 1976); Leo Orleans, *Health Policies and Services in China, 1974* (Washington, D.C.: U.S. Government Printing Office, 1974); and Victor W. Sidel and Ruth Sidel, *Serve the People: Observations on Medicine in the People's Republic of China* (Boston: Beacon Press, 1974), and "The Health Care Delivery System of the People's Republic of China," in Kenneth Newell, ed., *Health by the People* (Geneva: World Health Organization, 1975).

Collections of articles by specialists on medicine in China or by recent visitors to China include books published by the Fogarty International Center, National Institutes of Health, Bethesda, Maryland: Joseph R. Quinn, ed., *Medicine and Public Health in the People's Republic of China,* DHEW Publication no. (NIH) 72–67 (1972); Joseph R. Quinn, ed., *China Medicine As We Saw It,* DHEW Publication no. (NIH) 75–684, (1974); and Arthur Kleinman, Peter Kunstadter, E. Russell Alexander, and James L. Gale, eds., *Medicine in Chinese Cultures: Comparative Studies of Health Care in Chinese and Other Societies,* DHEW Publication no. (NIH) 75–653 (1975), particularly the chapter by H. Jack Geiger, "Health Care in the People's Republic of China: Implications for the United States," pp. 713–25. Collections published by the Macy Foundation include Myron E. Wegman, Tsung-yi Lin, and Elizabeth F. Purcell, eds. *Public Health in the People's Republic of China,* (1973); and John Z. Bowers and Elizabeth F. Purcell, eds., *Medicine and Society in China* (1974). An extensive annotated bibliography was prepared by S. Akhtar, *Health Care in the People's Republic of China: A Bibliography with Abstracts* (Ottawa: International Development Research Centre, 1975).

There is extensive material on the history of medicine in China. Joseph Needham's monumental, multivolume work, *Science and Civilization in China* (Cambridge: Cambridge University Press, 1954–70) is too detailed for most general readers, but some parts have been summarized in his book *The Grand Titration: Science and Society in*

East and West (London: George Allen & Unwin, 1969). Aspects of the history of traditional Chinese medicine are discussed in Ralph C. Croizier, *Traditional Medicine in Modern China* (Cambridge, Mass.: Harvard University Press, 1968); Pierre Huard and Ming Wong, *Chinese Medicine* (New York: McGraw-Hill Book Co., 1968); Stephen Palos, *The Chinese Art of Healing* (New York: Bantam Books, 1972); and Ilsa Veith's translation of and commentary on *The Yellow Emperor's Classic of Internal Medicine* (Berkeley: University of California Press, 1972).

The introduction of Western medicine is described by John Z. Bowers, *Western Medicine in a Chinese Palace: Peking Union Medical College, 1917–1951* (New York: Josiah Macy, Jr., Foundation, 1972), which includes the quotations from Lockhart (p. 4), Wu Lien-teh (p. 25), Eliot (p. 33), and Hume (p. 74). Hume's own experiences in China are described in Edward H. Hume, *Doctors East, Doctors West: An American Physician's Life in China* (New York: W. W. Norton & Co., 1946). Bertrand Russell's characterization of the work of Americans in China is in his cogent analysis, *The Problem of China* (London: George Allen & Unwin, 1922), p. 221. The recollections of Shanghai are those of W. A. Scott, "China Revisted by an Old China Hand," *Eastern Horizon* 5 (June 1966): 34–40.

A detailed analysis of the development of health policy in China since 1949 is presented by David M. Lampton, *Health, Conflict and the Chinese Political System* (Ann Arbor: University of Michigan Center for Chinese Studies, 1974). The relationship of medical care to ideology is explored by G. Gibson, "Chinese Medical Practice and the Thoughts of Chairman Mao," *Social Science and Medicine* 6 (February 1972): 67–93.

The campaign against schistosomiasis has been described by Leo A. Orleans and Richard P. Suttmeier, "The Mao Ethic and Environmental Quality," *Science* 170 (December 11, 1970): 1173–6.

Further material on the barefoot doctor may be found in Victor W. Sidel, "The Barefoot Doctors of the People's Republic of China," *New England Journal of Medicine* 286 (June 15, 1972): 1292–9; Virginia Li Wang, "Training of the Barefoot Doctor in the People's Republic of China: From Prevention to Curative Service," *International Journal of Health Services* 5, no. 3 (1975): 475–88; P. K. New and M. L. New, "Health Care in the People's Republic of China: The Barefoot Doctor," *Inquiry* 12 (June 1975): 103–13. Urban health-care services are described in Ruth Sidel, *Families of Fengsheng: Urban Life in China* (Baltimore: Penguin Books, 1974). Child health care was reviewed in 1973 by the Chinese Medical Association in *Child Health Care in New China,* reprinted in the *American Journal of Chinese Medicine* 2 (1974): 149–58, and by Joseph D. Wray, "Child Care in the People's Republic of China: 1973," *Pediatrics* 55 (April 1975): 539–50. Information on population control and family planning in China is given in Leo A. Orleans, *Every Fifth Child: The Population of China* (Stanford, Calif.: Stanford University Press, 1972); C. Djerassi, "Chinese Achievement in Fertility Control," *Bulletin of the Atomic Scientists* 30 (June 1974): 17–24; Ruth Sidel, *Women and Child Care in China: A Firsthand Report* (Baltimore: Penguin Books, 1973); and Han Suyin, "Family Planning in China," in Phyllis T. Piotrow, ed., *Population and Family Planning in the People's Republic of China* (New York: Victor-Bostrom Fund and Population Crisis Committee, 1971), pp. 16–21, from which her quotation is taken.

The financing of health care in China is analyzed in T. Hu, "Financing and Economic Efficiency of Rural Health Services in the People's Republic of China," *International Journal of Health Services* 6, no. 2 (1976): 239–49, and C. P. Wen and C. W. Hays, "Health Care Financing in China," *Medical Care* 14 (March 1976): 241–54. The official Chinese statement in 1963 is from *For the Health of the People* (Peking: Foreign Languages Press, 1963), pp. 2–3.

Chapter 6. Past and Present

Further material on the history of the American medical-care system can be found in Rosemary Stevens, *American Medicine and the Public Interest* (New Haven, Conn.: Yale University Press, 1971); Richard H. Shryock, *Medicine and Society in America: 1660–1860* (Ithaca, N.Y.: Cornell University Press, 1962); Joseph F. Kett, *The Formation of the American Medical Profession: The Role of Institutions, 1780–1860* (New Haven, Conn.: Yale University Press, 1968); John Duffy, *The Healers: The Rise of the Medical Establishment* (New York: McGraw-Hill Book Co., 1976); George Rosen, *From Medical Police to Social Medicine: Essays on the History of Health Care* (New York: Science History Publications, 1974); and George Rosen, *Preventive Medicine in the United States, 1900–1975* (New York: Prodist, 1975).

Information on Native American medicine can be found in Virgil

J. Vogel, *American Indian Medicine* (Norman: University of Oklahoma Press, 1970). The Winthrop statement of principles, John Smith's account of Jamestown, and William Douglass's letter on smallpox are reprinted in *The Annals of America* (Chicago: Encyclopedia Britannica, 1968), 1: 109–15, 21–31, 348–50. A detailed history and analysis of the development and organization of utopian communities in the United States can be found in Rosabeth Moss Kanter, *Commitment and Community: Communes and Utopias in Sociological Perspective* (Cambridge, Mass.: Harvard University Press, 1974). The efforts of the Puritan immigrants to create an ideal society are described and analyzed by Kenneth A. Lockridge, *A New England Town: The First Hundred Years* (New York: W. W. Norton & Co., 1970). Max Weber's analysis of the "Protestant Ethic" can be found in his book *The Protestant Ethic and the Spirit of Capitalism* (New York: Charles Scribner's Sons, 1958). The story of Thomas Wynne is told in Lewis Meier, *Early Pennsylvania Medicine* (Boyertown, Penn.: Gilbert Printing Co., 1976). The roles of Anne Hutchinson, Dr. Primus, and other "irregular" practitioners are discussed in Barbara Ehrenreich and Deirdre English, *Witches, Midwives and Nurses: A History of Women Healers* (Old Westbury, N.Y.: Feminist Press, 1973). Cotton Mather's comments on the treatment of measles are quoted in Duffy, *The Healers*, p. 35. Washington's order to inoculate the Continental Army was reported in *200 Years of Health and Medicine in the United States* (New York: Metropolitan Life Insurance Co., 1976). The material on public health in New York City is from John Duffy, "Public Health in New York City in the Revolutionary Period," *Journal of the American Medical Association* 236 (July 5, 1976): 47–51. The estimate of the number of physicians in the colonies at the time of the Revolution may be found in *200 Years of Health and Medicine in the United States.*

A discussion of the popular health movement is presented in Ehrenreich and English, *Witches, Midwives and Nurses,* and in Richard H. Shryock, *Medicine in America: Historical Essays* (Baltimore: Johns Hopkins University Press, 1966). The conflict between health and property rights is discussed by Julian McCaull, "Pursuit of Property," *Environment* 18 (July–August 1976): 17–31.

A history of the role of the AMA is given in James G. Burrow, *AMA: Voice of American Medicine* (Baltimore: Johns Hopkins University Press, 1963). Recent activities of the AMA are described in Elton Rayack, *Professional Power and American Medicine: The Eco-*

nomics of the American Medical Association (Cleveland, Ohio: World Publishing Co., 1967), and Richard Harris, *A Sacred Trust* (Baltimore: Penguin Books, 1969). Abraham Flexner's *Medical Education in the United States and Canada,* published by the Carnegie Foundation in 1910, has been reprinted (New York: Arno Press, 1972). The final report of the Committee on the Costs of Medical Care, *Medical Care for the American People* (Chicago: University of Chicago Press, 1932), has been reprinted by Arno Press and *The New York Times,* New York, 1972. An analysis of the failure to enact compulsory health insurance in the United States during the 1930s is provided in Daniel S. Hirshfield, *The Lost Reform: The Campaign for Compulsory Health Insurance in the United States from 1932 to 1943* (Cambridge, Mass.: Harvard University Press, 1970), and the problems in other forms of health insurance are discussed in Sylvia A. Law, *Blue Cross: What Went Wrong?* 2nd ed. (New Haven, Conn.: Yale University Press, 1976).

Material on the neighborhood health centers of the 1960s may be found in D. I. Zwick, "Some Accomplishments and Findings of Neighborhood Health Centers," *Milbank Memorial Fund Quarterly* 50 (October 1972): 387–420. The Martin Luther King Health Center in the Bronx is described in William B. Lloyd and Harold B. Wise, "The Montefiore Experience," *Bulletin of the New York Academy of Medicine* 44 (November 1968): 1353–62.

The Mound Bayou Health Center in Mississippi is described in H. Jack Geiger, "A Health Center in Mississippi: A Case Study in Social Medicine," in Lawrence Corey, S. E. Saltman, and M. F. Epstein, eds., *Medicine in a Changing Society* (St. Louis: C. V. Mosby Co., 1972), pp. 157–67. A description of the community development effort which grew out of the Mound Bayou Health Center may be found in Herbert Black, *People and Plows Against Hunger: Self-Help Experiment in a Rural Community* (Boston: Marlborough House, 1975).

A detailed analysis of the impact of the Nixon years on medical services is given in Victor W. Sidel, "Medical Care: Playing Politics with Health," in Alan Gartner, Colin Greer, and Frank Riessman, eds., *What Nixon Is Doing to Us* (New York: Harper & Row, 1973), pp. 58–83. An account of the passage of the legislation creating the National Health Service Corps is presented in Eric Redman, *The Dance of Legislation* (New York: Simon & Schuster, 1973).

The rapidity of social change is described by Alvin Toffler, *Future*

Shock (New York: Bantam Books, 1970); his comment on mobility is on p. 75. Population distribution in the United States is estimated regularly in *Current Population Reports,* ser. P-20.

Herbert Gans's analysis of inner-city residents can be found in his chapter, "Urbanism and Suburbanism As Ways of Life: A Re-evaluation of Definitions," in Arnold Rose, ed., *Human Behavior and Social Process* (Boston: Houghton Mifflin Co., 1962).

Much of the material on current patterns of urbanization in the United States and specifically the quotation from the Commission on Crimes of Violence set up by Lyndon Johnson was taken from Brian J. L. Berry, *The Human Consequences of Urbanization* (New York: St. Martin's Press, 1973), p. 54. The explanation of contemporary migration from the cities to the suburbs is given by Berry, p. 51.

The quotation from Tocqueville is on p. 536 of *Democracy in America* (Garden City, N.Y.: Doubleday Anchor Books, 1969). The data on geographic mobility are given in Larry H. Lang and Celia G. Boertlein, *The Geographical Mobility of Americans: An International Comparison* (Washington, D.C.: Bureau of the Census, 1976).

Ernest Becker's analysis of the meaning of death in U.S. society can be found in his book *The Denial of Death* (New York: Free Press, 1973), p. ix.

Chapter 7. Proposals and Prospects

Recommendations for initial, minimal steps in preventive medicine were prepared by a series of task forces sponsored by the John E. Fogarty International Center for Advanced Study in the Health Sciences of the National Institutes of Health and the American College of Preventive Medicine, and published in *Preventive Medicine USA* (New York: Prodist, 1976). The Task Force on Environmental Health Services presented recommendations in the areas of occupational safety and health; housing; water, food and nutrition; air contamination; injuries; physical agents; factors in production of cancer and genetic defects; and chronic and degenerative diseases. Approaches to dealing with the apparent conflict between prevention of environmental pollution and avoiding greater unemployment are discussed by Barry Commoner, *The Poverty of Power* (New York: Alfred

A. Knopf, 1976). Other recommendations in the area of occupational health and safety can be found in Jeanne M. Stellman and Susan M. Daum, *Work Is Dangerous to Your Health: A Handbook of Health Hazards in the Workplace and What You Can Do About Them* (New York: Vintage Books, 1971). Recommendations in the area of health education, made by the Task Force on Health Promotion and Consumer Health Protection, are also published in Anne R. Somers, ed., *Promoting Health: Consumer Education and National Policy* (Germantown, Md.: Aspen Systems Corp., 1976). Recommendations in the area of primary and secondary prevention for individuals are made by the Task Force on Prevention in Personal Health Services.

The comment by H. L. Mencken was supplied by Michael Halberstam.

Recommendations on the collection of data independent of race were made by Milton Terris, "Desegregating Health Statistics," *American Journal of Public Health* 63 (June 1973): 477–80.

Discussions of the various forms of health insurance and their relationship to a national health service may be found in T. S. Bodenheimer, "The Hoax of National Health Insurance," *American Journal of Public Health* 62 (October 1972): 1324–7; Milton Terris, "The Need for a National Health Program," *Bulletin of the New York Academy of Medicine* 48 (January 1972): 24–31; Eveline M. Burns, *Health Services for Tomorrow* (New York: Dunellen Publishing Co., 1973); Karen Davis, *National Health Insurance: Benefits, Costs, and Consequences* (Washington, D.C.: Brookings Institution, 1975); and M. I. Roemer and S. J. Axelrod, "A National Health Service and Social Security," *American Journal of Public Health* 67 (May 1977): 462–5. Copies of proposals for a national health service may be obtained from the Committee for a National Health Service, Box 2125, New York, N.Y. 10001, and from the office of Congressman Ronald Dellums, Washington, D.C. The statement by the four past presidents of the American Public Health Association is also available from the Committee for a National Health Service. Resolutions of the American Public Health Association on the issue were published in the January 1977 issue of the *American Journal of Public Health,* vol. 67, pp. 84 and 86.

Much of the discussion of the control of the quality of medical care originally appeared in Victor W. Sidel, "Quality for Whom? Effects of Professional Responsibility for Quality of Health Care on Equity," *Bulletin of the New York Academy of Medicine* 52 (January 1976):

164–76. Reviews of other aspects of this topic may be found in A. Donabedian, *A Guide to Medical Care Administration II: Medical Care Appraisal—Quality and Utilization* (Washington, D.C.: American Public Health Association, 1969); R. H. Brook and F. A. Appel, "Quality of Care Assessment: Choosing a Method for Peer Review," *New England Journal of Medicine* 288 (June 21, 1973): 1323–29. The statement on means and ends is from C. J. Hitch, *The Economics of Defense in the Nuclear Age* (Cambridge, Mass.: Harvard University Press, 1960). The quotation from Frantz Fanon is in *A Dying Colonialism* (New York: Grove Press, 1967), p. 9; that from Mao Tsetung, in *Four Essays on Philosophy* (Peking: Foreign Languages Press, 1966), p. 8; and that from Thomas Jefferson, in "A Letter to William Charles Jarvis," September 28, 1820, quoted in John Bartlett, *Familiar Quotations* (Boston: Little, Brown & Co., 1955), p. 375b.

The numerous recent sources on the self-help movement include Lowell S. Levin, Alfred H. Katz, and Erik Holst, eds., *Self-Care: Lay Initiatives in Health* (New York: Prodist, 1976); Alfred H. Katz and Eugene I. Bender, eds., *The Strength in Us: Self-help Groups in the Modern World* (New York: Franklin Watts, 1976); *Self-help and Health: A Report,* New Human Services Institute, Queens College–CUNY, September 1976, particularly Alan Gartner and Frank Riessman, "Health Care in a Technological Age," from which the quotation on the number of self-help groups in Massachusetts is taken (p. 21); and a special self-help issue of *Social Policy* (September–October 1976), particularly Victor W. Sidel and Ruth Sidel, "Beyond Coping," pp. 67–9.

The questions raised by the director-general of the World Health Organization may be found in H. Mahler, "Tomorrow's Medicine and Tomorrow's Doctors," *WHO Chronicle* 31 (February 1977): 60–2.

The "lifeboat" ethic is presented by Garrett Hardin, "Living on a Lifeboat," *Bioscience* 24 (October 1974): 561–8, and discussed by Daniel Callahan, "Doing Well by Doing Good," *Hastings Center Report* 4 (December 1974): 1–4. WHO's new position is stated in Kenneth Newell, ed., *Health by the People* (Geneva: World Health Organization, 1975), and in V. Djukanovic and E. P. Mach, eds., *Alternative Approaches to Meeting Basic Health Needs in Developing Countries* (Geneva: World Health Organization, 1975). A recent discussion by the director-general of WHO of the implications of the United Nations resolution on a "New Economic Order" was published in H. Mahler, "WHO and the New Economic Order," *WHO Chronicle* 30 (June 1976): 215–22.

The arguments in opposition to a right to health care were analyzed by Victor W. Sidel in "The Right to Health Care: An International Perspective," presented at the Interdisciplinary Conference on Bioethics and Human Rights, Long Island University, to be published as a chapter in Bertram Bandman and Elsie Bandman, eds., *Bioethics and Human Rights: A Reader for Health Professionals* (Boston: Little, Brown & Co., in press). The quotation from Charles Fried is from "Equality and Rights in Medical Care," *Hastings Center Report* 6 (February 1976): 29–34. The Robert Sade quotation may be found in his article "Medical Care As a Right: A Refutation," *New England Journal of Medicine* 285 (December 2, 1971): 1288–92.

The statement by Virchow is quoted in Henry Sigerist, *On the Sociology of Medicine,* ed. Milton I. Roemer (New York: MD Publications, 1960), p. 379.

INDEX

abortion laws, 18
accidents: as cause of death, 19, 20; prevention of, 48–9
acupuncture, 190
addiction, 290
age and aging. *See* elderly people
age-specific death rates, 188; international comparisons, 10–12; Swedish, 111. *See also* life expectancy
Alabama, 60, 68
Al-Anon, 290
Alaska, 241
Alateen, 290
alcohol and alcoholism, 20, 49, 50, 170; Swedish, 111
Alexander II (Russia), 163
Algeria, 289
ambulance attendants, 79
ambulatory care, 53, 55, 56, 58, 259, 286; British, 130, 139; Swedish, 119–20, 122, 123–4, 126
American College of Surgeons, 5
American Dilemma, The (Myrdal), *xviii*
American health-care and medical-care system. *See* U. S. health-care and medical-care system
American health status, 7–8, 9–27; death rates and life expectancy, 10–21; disability rates, 23–5; illness rates, 21–3; malnutrition and poor physical fitness, 26. *See also* United States
American Hospital Association, 239

American Medical Association, 87, 99, 228, 234, 237, 245, 246, 281, 296
American Public Health Association, 283
American society: family unit, 252; fear of death in, 254–5; geographic mobility, 251–2; poverty in, 253–4. *See also* United States
American Statistical Society, 230
anemia, 74
anesthesia, 5, 7, 227, 234
anesthesiologists, 77
antibiotics, 7, 201, 234; dangers of, 73–4; marketing of, 101–2. *See also* drugs; medication
antielitism, 266, 292
antisepsis, 227
apothecaries, 134–5, 224
Appalachia, 60, 62
Argentina, 23, 102
Armed Services, 56
arthritis, 7, 25, 45, 67, 92, 102
aspirin, 102
Association of American Medical Colleges, 57, 296
asthma, 7
Australia, *xxxiv,* 14, 16, 252
automobile accidents, 20, 48
automobile industry: health insurance, 36

Baltimore, 23, 24
barber-surgeons, 224
barefoot doctors, 177, 190, 204–7,

peptic ulcer, 161
Peter the Great (Russia), 165, 184
pharmaceutical industry, 55, 154.
  See also drug companies
pharmacists, 53, 64, 79; Chinese,
  200; income, 43; Soviet, 171,
  175–6. *See also* health workers
Philadelphia, 225, 226, 239
Philippines, 103
physical examination, 50–1
physical fitness, 26–27
physicians, 262, 267; authority of,
  79–81; British, 130–44; Chinese,
  traditional, 191–2; colonial American, 223, 224–6; complaints of, 4;
  ethics, 88; foreign, in U. S., 98–
  101; freedom of choice for, 142–3;
  home visits, 90; hospital based, 58,
  63; income, 42–3, 82, 84; incorporated, 42; maldistribution of,
  60–64; malpractice of, 77–78;
  Medicaid and, 63–64; nineteenth-
  century, 227–9; obstetrician-
  gynecologists, 42; pediatricians,
  21, 91, 77, 122, 179; primary-care,
  53, 58, 86; professional supremacy
  of, 79–81, 88, 127; psychiatrists,
  42; public confidence in, 8–9; public expectations of, 90–91; race, sex
  and economic status of, 82; scientific emphasis of, 235; selection
  and training patterns, 263–4;
  shortages of, 237; Soviet, 159, 161,
  162–3, 170, 174–9; specialization
  trend, 58; surgeons, 42, 75–77,
  224, 226; Swedish, 113, 114, 116,
  120, 123, 127; training and practice of, 57–58; women, 159, 166,
  172, 175, 178–9, 223, 225, 228; *See
  also* general practitioners; medical
  schools
physician's assistant programs, 86–
  88
Physicians Forum, 282
physician's union, 88–89
physician visits: by age and income,
  64–67; American vs. Swedish, 122;
  by race, 67–68

pertussis. *See* whooping cough
Pirogov, N. I., 163
Pirogov Society, 170, 234
plague, 197, 202
pneumonic plague, 194
poisoning, 19
Poland, 23, 24
poliomyelitis, 8, 48, 206
polyclinics, 178, 185
poor people, 22, 231, 232, 238,
  253–4; access to medical care, 5–6,
  63–7, 136–7, 162, 235–6; disability
  rates of, 25; health insurance for,
  38; illness rates of, 22, 47–8; infant
  mortality rates, 17; physician visits
  per year, 63–67; rate of checkups
  of, 51
popular health movement, 227
populist movement, 227
practical nurses, 79, 84
pregnancy. *See* maternal mortality;
  prenatal care
prenatal care, *xxii–xxiii;* New York
  study, 50
prepaid group practice, 275–6
prescriptions: unnecessary, 73–4
President's Task Force on Manpower Conservation, 26
preventive medicine, 44–52, 58, 103,
  178, 258, 260, 275, 285; accident
  prevention, 48–9; British, 139,
  144–5; checkups, 50–52; Chinese,
  191–2, 198, 199–200, 204, 205;
  habit and life-style changes, 49–
  50; immunization programs, 47–8;
  prenatal care, 50; primary, 47–50;
  screening programs, 50–2; Soviet,
  160–1, 179–80; Swedish approach,
  121–2; tertiary, 47, 52
primary care, 53, 54, 87, 91, 103, 178,
  261–2; British, 129, 130, 138, 139,
  144–5; community-based, 258;
  defined, 53; rural Soviet, 182–3;
  training for, 152–3
Primitive Physic (Wesley), 223
Professional Standards Review Organizations, 247, 283
prostheses, 90

About the Authors

Victor W. Sidel, M.D., is Chairman of the Department of Social Medicine at Montefiore Hospital and Medical Center, and Professor of Community Health at the Albert Einstein College of Medicine in New York. He has studied at first hand the health-care systems of over a dozen nations and serves as a frequent consultant to the World Health Organization.

Ruth Sidel is a graduate of Wellesley College and Boston University School of Social Work. She is the author of *Women and Child Care in China* and *Families of Fengsheng: Urban Life in China,* and coauthor with Victor Sidel of *Serve the People: Observations on Medicine in the People's Republic of China.*